Hormonal Timing: Female Fitness EVOLVED!
by BuffMother!

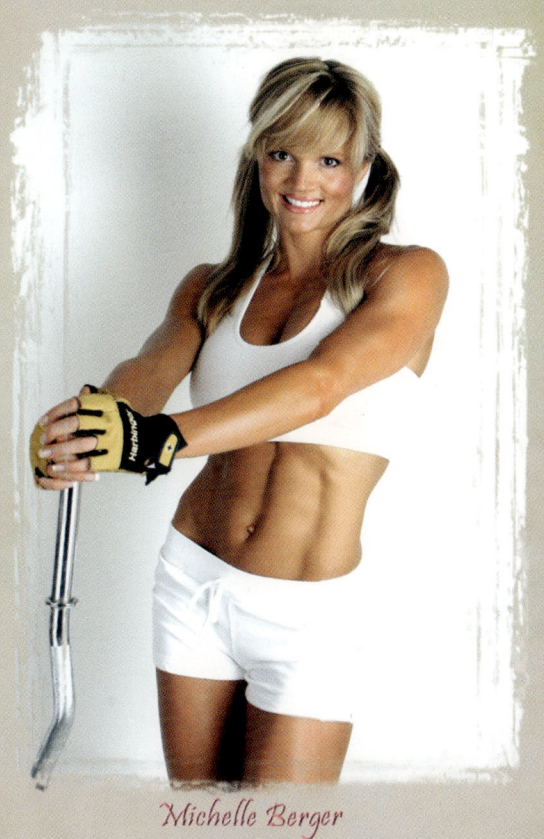

Michelle Berger
aka BuffMother!

Generational Health Publications
1401 S. Walton Blvd. Ste. 9-127
Bentonville, AR 72712

Hormonal Timing by BuffMother!
Female Fitness Evolved

Copyright © 2007 by Michelle Berger

All rights reserved. Printed in the United States of America. No part of this book may be used or reproduced without written permission except in the case of personal journaling, and brief quotations embodied in articles and reviews. This book is intended for healthy adults, age 18 and over. This book expresses the author's opinions and is solely for informational and educational purposes and is not medical advice. Please consult with a medical or health professional before you begin any new exercise, nutrition or supplementation program or if you have questions about your health. The testimonies featured are unpaid and represent examples of what can be accomplished over time through an integrated system of exercise, nutrition, supplementation and mental strategies. As individuals differ their results will differ, even when following similar methods. The statements made within this book have not been evaluated by the Food and Drug Administration. BuffMother LLC and Generational Health Publications LLC do not accept any responsibility for injury sustained as a result of following the advice or suggestions contained within the content of this book.

For information about permissions to reproduce selections from this book, or to purchase books for educational, business or sales promotional use, please write:
Generational Health Publications
1401 S. Walton Blvd. Ste. 9-127
Bentonville, AR 72712

Library of Congress Cataloging- in Publications Data
Berger, Michelle
Hormonal Timing by BuffMother!: Female Fitness Evolved

Library of Congress Control Number: 2007908662

International Standard Book Number: 978-0-9800363-0-5
FIRST EDITION
Printed in the USA

Published by Generational Health Publications
Design by Emily McArthur
Photos by Emily McArthur, D. Brady, Chris Bray
Edit by Gina Wagner & Darcie Arent
Graphic contributions by Darcie Arent

Join BuffMother! online at www.BuffMother.com

10 Secrets to Success

I am constantly being asked questions like, "How did you do it?" and "What's your secret?" I have literally received THOUSANDS of e-mails asking me these types of questions! Everyone is looking for a fast and easy system that yields incredible results, right? Well, over the past few years, I have had the opportunity to work with hundreds of women and together, we have identified 10 secrets that will guarantee success. I refer to these theses secrets as the "10 Foundations" because it is absolutely impossible to fail if you are willing to simply build your fitness/lifestyle upon the proper foundations. I truly believe the "10 Foundations" are the fastest, easiest way to revolutionize your body, life and legacy! The cool thing is that if you were to implement only 1 of the "10 Foundations," you would reap great benefits. This book will teach you exactly how to apply all of these foundations through the use of 10 simple and effective "Success Tools." My dramatic, continual results are due to the fact that I relentlessly follow these foundations and they have become my lifestyle. Over the past 4 years, I have taught them to private clients from all over the world and they ALWAYS work! Please, test them for yourself! You will be amazed! And remember~ I will be here beside you every step of the way!

From Fluff...

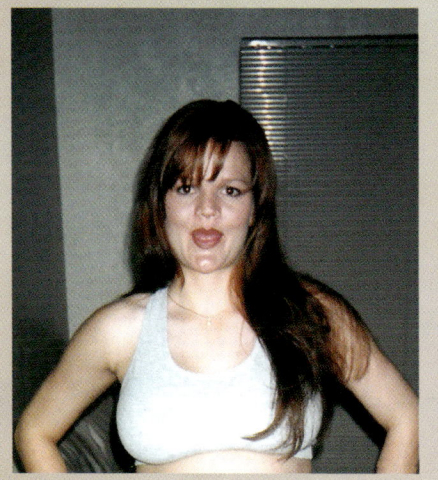

...to BUFF!

This was me before I had children...

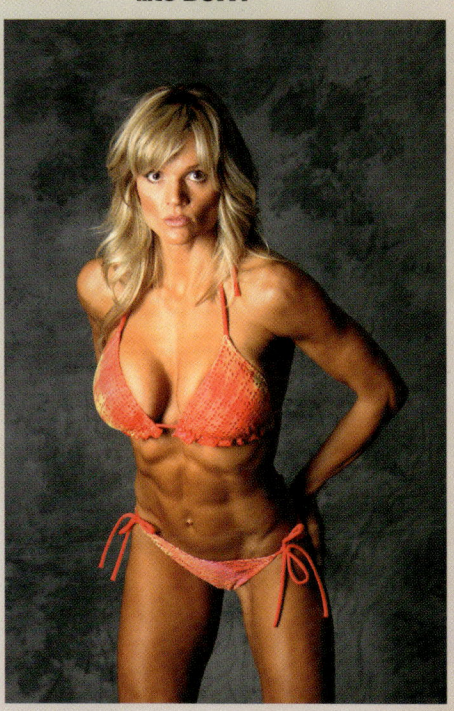

...and this is me now, after 4!

How to use this book~

1. Read <u>ALL</u> of it. Take notes and get engaged.

2. Be inspired by the great testimonies from women just like you.

3. Learn and believe in the 10 Foundations.

4. Implement each Foundation's Success Tool into your life.

5. Build momentum by your small choices; the Foundations Success Journal will help keep you on track to success.

6. Plug into the Rally Room: the world's best support system! ~ FOR WOMEN ONLY

This book is dedicated to:

~Every woman who has a deep down desire to improve her life.~

THANKS TEAM BUFFMOTHER!:

Ladies, thank you for your constant excitement, drive and determination to be your BEST!! Team BuffMother! is the most successful team of women that I have ever seen. We share a bond that can never be broken and I know we will strengthen and encourage each other forever. I would especially like to thank you for welcoming every new team member with open arms. You are truly changing lives all over the world. I am honored to have women like you in my life!

A special thanks to my husband, Travis:

Thank you for making me "BuffMother!" For without you and our four kids I'd just be "Michelle." Your unconditional love and continual encouragement have meant the world to me. Thanks for teaching me to <u>believe!!</u> I will love you FOREVER!!

And to my kids:

Thanks for being so cute, sweet, patient, and loving. Your laughter, hugs, and kisses are what fuel me to create a legacy you will admire.

Table of Contents

I. IF I Can Do It, You Can Too!
- Blood, Sweat, Tears and Diapers
- Key Terms
- Seeing is Believing
- Darcie's Testimony

II. Female Fitness Evolved
- Eureka!
- Lisa's Testimony
- Foundation #1: Realize That You Are in a Battle!
- Hormones Control Your Diet and Fitness Success!
- Success Tool #1- Identify HIF Patterns
- Doctor Testimonials

III. Harness The Power of Your Hormones
- Foundation #2: Hormonal Timing
- HOW TO Apply Hormonal Timing To Your Life
- Success Tool #2- Buffing and Boosting
- How Buffing and Boosting Work Together
- Leslie's Testimony

IV. Train Your BRAIN
- Foundation #3: You Must BELIEVE!
- Success Tool #3- Doubt Crushers
- Julie's Testimony
- Foundation #4: PMA- All The Way BABY!
- Success Tool #4- Focus On Solutions
- How to Create Exponential Energy
- Foundation #5: Energize Others
- Success Tool #5- The Rally Room
- Cara's Testimony
- Evaluate your "WHY"

IV. Train Your BRAIN (cont.)
- Foundation #6: Your Strong WHY- Your Legacy!
- Success Tool #6- The 24 Hour Legacy Test
- Foundation #7: Momentum!
- Success Tool #7- "5 Minute MoJo"
- Generational Health Testimonies: Jenn, April

V. Nuts and Bolts for ACTION
- 7 BuffMother Basics
- Foundation #8: Plan Of Attack! (POA)
- Success Tool #8- Step By Step Illustrated Exercise Plan
- BuffMotherobics! Interval Training
- Foundation #9: Your Diet is Simple
- Success Tool #9- The 5-4-3-2-1 Diet
- Foundation #10: Measuring Success
- Success Tool #10- Foundations Success Journal

BONUS Section:
- BONUS: Hormonal Timing SEX- It Will Blow Your Mind!

Appendixes
A. Success Tool #1-Identify HIF Patterns
B. Starting Statistics, Measurements, and Pictures
C. Guideline for Progression of Workouts
D. Sample Diet Menu
E. Success Tool #10-Foundations Success Journal
F. Other Resources and Products by BuffMother!

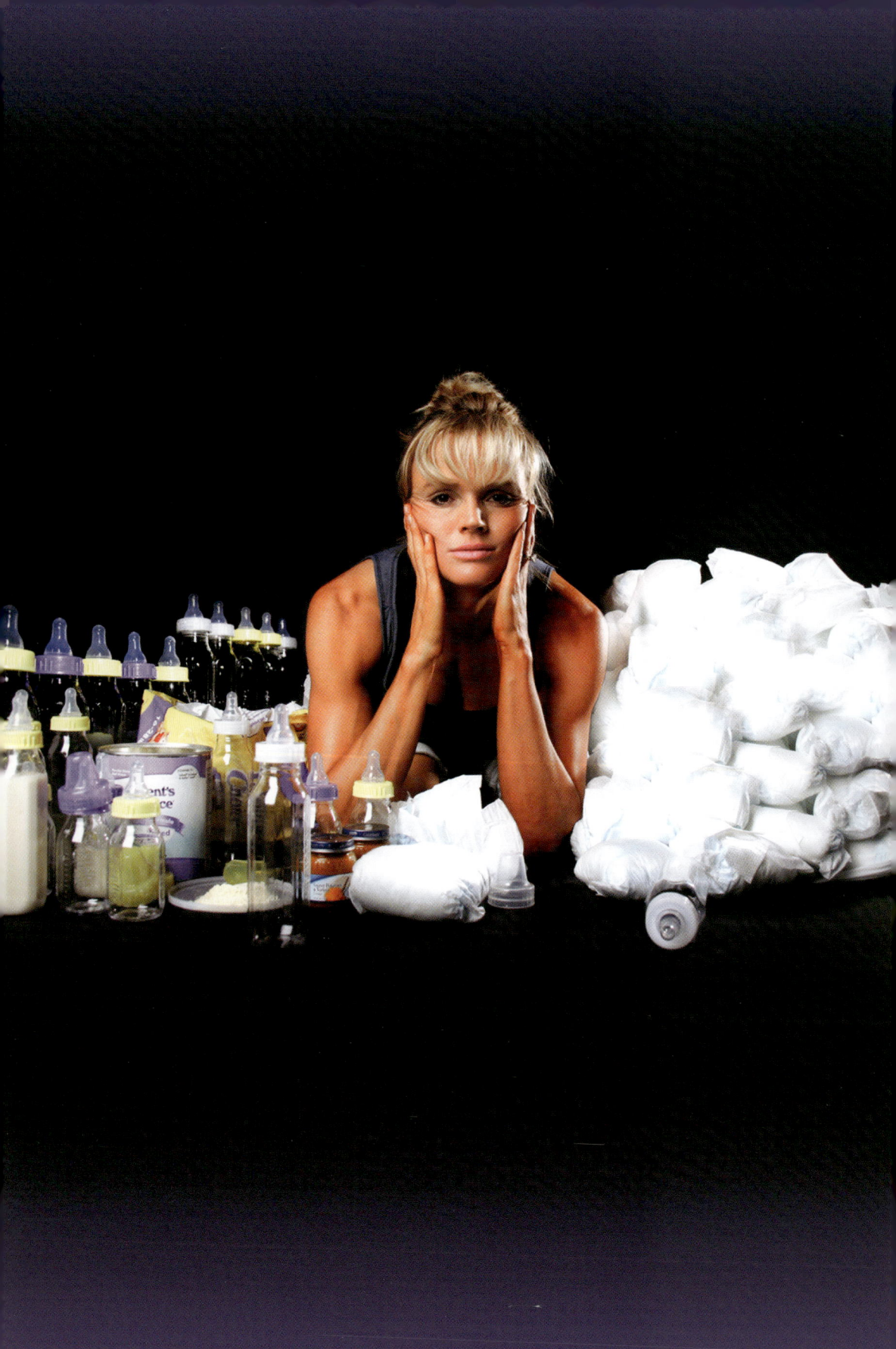

section 1

If I can do it...

...You can too!

Blood, Sweat, Tears, and Diapers

I'll never forget how I felt when I noticed cellulite on my body for the first time. I was still in high school and worked at the local bakery. It was bikini season in Minnesota and time to go to the lake. However, my bikini from the previous year wasn't exactly fitting. When I looked in the mirror I noticed cellulite everywhere! My butt, stomach, back and legs were covered with it and I was shocked! I guess eating doughnuts hand over fist all winter had caught up with me. I was crushed! Luckily, track season was just around the corner and I was young enough to get pretty good results from running and cutting back on the doughnuts. It was this experience that made me choose to study Exercise Science and Nutrition in college. I was never going to let this ugly stuff form my body again. Little did I know that the battle was just beginning.

I worked hard in college and learned everything I could about exercise and nutrition. I was awarded a track scholarship which helped me to keep very fit and active. However, all the running was taking a toll on my body. I was often injured and eventually I developed a knee problem that surgery couldn't fix. My 3-year collegiate track career was over and I was forced to spend my last year of college sitting on the sidelines.

After college, I began working in Dallas for a company that built new home developments. They were developing an area on the outskirts of Dallas and they wanted me to be the community fitness director. I was very excited to put my education to use. However, since the homes were just being built, I was asked to perform other management duties until the development was finished. This meant long hours sitting behind a desk and unfortunately eating way too many Otis Spunkmeyer cookies! It wasn't long until my clothes started to feel a little snug. In fact, I started to gain a lot of weight very quickly! Obesity is prevalent among the women in my family and it wanted to afflict me. I decided to declare war on my fat and get in tip-top physical condition. I was on a mission.

I began to employ everything my expensive college education had taught me. It was a constant struggle for me to find a way to get results. I worked out harder, doing an hour of cardio 6 days a week and I still got bigger!!! I was hungry all the time and couldn't control my carbohydrate cravings. I was banging my head against the wall. Fitness advice was everywhere, but I was more confused than ever. The "experts" said, try to do at least an hour of cardio every day and if possible do two and cut the fat in your diet. Eat low fat and plenty of carbohydrates for energy. But their advice wasn't working. I was getting fatter, and once again covered with cellulite. I thought I was doing everything right so I began to question my education and the "experts." I questioned everything! Did anyone have a solution for me???

I experimented with every popular diet and exercise program on the market. I think I tried them all: Atkins, South Beach, The Slim Fast Plan, etc. I did get results from some of them, but I couldn't stick to them and my body was not transforming into what I wanted. I would usually achieve a 5 pound loss and then after my willpower gave out, I gained it back (plus some). The programs that did yield results were impossible for me to stick to. I could barely last 2 weeks so how was I supposed to live the rest of my life? Not this way! I began losing hope of ever looking good in a bikini again. It was at this time that I received the shocking news that I was pregnant!

Goodbye Body, Hello Mommy

After the shock wore off, I was very excited about being a mother, but I was also sad that I had to give up my hope to ever have a great body again. I was always taught that once you have a baby your body will never be the same. "Your hips will never go back," people told me. "Say goodbye to your body and hello

If I can do it...YOU can too!

to motherhood." I tried to exercise and eat a healthful diet but my efforts were inconsistent at best and I soon gave up. I decided to welcome my new mommy role and the "mommy body" that came with it.

Soon after the birth of my son I started to exercise again. I did not have a car at the time so I walked everywhere pushing my precious baby boy in the stroller. I figured at least I could try to look good in clothes and went on a mission to get as skinny as possible. I basically went on a starvation diet. I drank coffee all day and then had one meal. I never ate more than 1000 calories a day. (Numerous Hollywood stars practice this same lifestyle). I did look OK in clothes, but I felt horrible! I was very undernourished and had no energy. At the time I didn't care how unhealthy this lifestyle was. I was just doing what I thought was necessary to be thin. When my son was almost 2, I decided to give strength training a try. I had been avoiding it like a plague over the past 6 years because I thought it would make me look bigger. My greatest fear was looking like a female bodybuilder! I found that strength training was much more enjoyable than doing cardio for hours, and better yet, I began to see changes in my body. However, my results were very short lived because that month I got some life-changing news...

Pure CHAOS

"You're pregnant again" were the words of my doctor. We were surprised for a second time! I was excited but very scared. I did not have enough energy for 2 kids. I had managed to do OK with one baby, but I was at my limit. Yet again, I tried to exercise, but it didn't last long. Three months of morning sickness combined with severe hip pain and pelvic pressure made me a fit-pregnancy failure once again! However, I did manage to strength train about twice a week until about 3 weeks before giving birth. Just that little bit of muscle building seemed to make a big difference in my body composition. It was at this point that I made a huge decision. I decided to go on a mission to prove it's possible to have an awesome body after having children. I knew plenty of mothers who looked decent in clothes, but I wanted to prove it's possible to have the best body of your life after children. I didn't know how I would do it but I was going to make it happen.

So what strategy did I choose to employ?? I went right back to my old habits; starvation and cardio!! Looking back, I realize that I was a scale addict! I was convinced that losing weight was the recipe for looking great. According to the scale, I should have been very happy, but I was miserable. I was always tired, and the only way to describe my body was "SKINNY FAT!"; I had lost the weight, but my body was still soft and flabby. I hated looking in the mirror because I looked horrible without clothes on. I began to realize that a body without any muscle tone is not an attractive site. I realized right then and there that I desperately needed to include a strength component to my fitness strategy.

I wanted to feel strong and energetic. I wanted to eat again, I wanted to add some youthful muscle to my withering "skinny fat" body, and more than anything I wanted to set a powerful example for my son and 6-month-old daughter. I was once again on a mission! However, it was very short lived because I suddenly became very ill. A trip to the drug store for a pregnancy test revealed the shocking news that I was already pregnant again!!

Completely Incapacitated

I was sick! This pregnancy was much different than the previous two. Something was horribly wrong! I couldn't even get out of bed. I had two small children to care for plus all the housework and I felt like I'd been hit by a bus. It didn't take long for the doctors to figure out the problem. I was seven weeks pregnant with twins!! The reason I felt so rotten was because I had double the hormones compared to a normal pregnancy. I could not believe the dramatic effect these added hormones had on me. This experience made me realize that hormones are incredibly powerful! This also led to my "eureka" moment, that HORMONES CONTROL EVERYTHING!! I developed an overwhelming curiosity to find out everything I could relevant to women and hormones. I didn't know it at the time but this revelation would soon change my life!

Wide Load Coming Through

I was advised by my doctor to gain at least 50 pounds during this pregnancy. I remember thinking to myself, "there is no way I can bounce back from that!" However, the health of my babies was unquestionably my primary concern, so I proceeded to pack on the pounds. I got big! I mean really big! At that point my mission to create my best body ever was completely out the window. My belly was so BIG and I was terrified because I knew I had never seen a mother of twins who didn't "look the part." I was on bed rest for the last month and spent the last 3 weeks at the hospital hooked up to machines as they pumped nasty drugs into me in an effort to stop labor until the babies were fully developed. One of the drugs they use is called "Mag" (Magnesium Sulfate) and that stuff was pure agony! Then my doctor decided it was time to deliver the babies by c-section due to their positioning. I know this sounds a little crazy but I asked him to make my incision as small as he could and below my bikini line if at all possible. I guess in the back of my mind I was still thinking of my "impossible mission." He obliged and I gave birth to two beautiful baby girls we named Tia and Layla.

Overwhelmed

My situation was very daunting to me. I had four children and the oldest was only 3 years old. At that time my life consisted of laundry, cooking, cleaning, grocery shopping, nursing, pumping, bottles, diapers and dealing with four screaming babies! My husband was working long hours and traveling extensively trying make enough money to support a family of six, so I was on my own with the kids much of the time. I was a wreck! The twins needed to be fed every two hours and it took me an hour to feed them. I was functioning on virtually no sleep and my body was stretched out, fat, saggy and very ugly.

My friends and family just nodded and tried to downplay my passion to get in shape again. It seemed like the more people I shared my "dream" with the more negative comments I faced. They would say I was wasting my time. "You can't do it after having all those kids, not with your crazy life." My friends would urge me, "Don't worry about it so much." Why shouldn't I worry about it?? I wasn't happy, healthy, confident, energetic, etc. I needed to find a way to be the woman I wanted to be. I desperately wanted to be an awesome mother and set a great example for my 3 girls and my son! I needed them to see me laugh, play, enjoy eating and enjoy my life. I wanted them to have the knowledge, belief and habits to be healthy and successful in life. I wanted to create a legacy of health and fitness in my family.

A "Hunch" Paid Off

Despite the discouragement from others, I was excited to attack the transformation process. My mission to create my "best body ever" was back on. My driving force was to establish a legacy of health and fitness for my family and to prove all the naysayers wrong. I wanted to lead my kids by example. I wanted boundless energy so I could play with my kids. I wanted my girls to see that true beauty starts **after** you have children. I was determined to end the cycle of ill health, disability, and obesity that exists throughout my family. By this time I had developed a theory of using the power of my natural hormonal fluctuations to get fit. I was 100 percent certain that my hormones held the key to my best body ever and now was the time to prove it!

I joined the gym when my twins were 5 months old and went back to what I knew had given me the best results in the past: strength training and intervals. I also began experimenting with diet, exercise and supplementation combinations according to my monthly cycle. In just a few months, my results were shocking! I could not believe it! My body quickly began to morph into exactly what I had wanted for the last 10 years. **Hormonal Timing was born!** Women began approaching me in the gym asking me to be their personal trainer. I wanted to help as many women as I could so I began working with several clients. I was so excited to see that they were seeing results like mine! I knew

If I can do it...YOU can too!

I was onto something huge and that Hormonal Timing would revolutionize women's fitness.

I wanted to see if my results were as impressive as I hoped they were. When my twins were only 13 months old, I really tested my results by entering a NPC, National Physique Committee, figure contest (basically a beauty pageant where you present yourself on a stage in front of thousands of people in both one-piece and two-piece, jewel adorned formal swimsuit). The judges score you on your overall beauty, stage presence, body symmetry and feminine muscle shape. Most of the other competitors were younger and did not have children, so I was very nervous about getting on stage with them in a bikini.

I was floored when the judges announced that I won! My belief in Hormonal Timing skyrocketed! This was real and nobody could argue with my results. I went on to win 5 figure titles that year. I had proven it is possible to look great after having children no matter what obstacles stand in the way.

My BuffMother! Mission Began

My hunger to help every woman in the world led me to start my website BuffMother.com. I feel it is my God-given mission to give hope to other women that are where I was…FRUSTRATED. I want women to know that they have the choice to take control of their bodies and lives and establish a legacy of health and fitness in their home. I've used the internet to tell my story and share what I learned "in the trenches." I want women to realize that their life as a desirable, vibrant, successful and confident woman does not have to end once they become a mother. Being a mother is a component of who we are, but doesn't have to be our only identity. In order for us to be a happy person and best mother possible, we need to take time to nurture ourselves. Living your dream is possible!

"Hormonal Timing is the Future of Female Diet, Fitness, and Supplementation."

If I can do it…YOU can too!

Key Terms in this book:

Boosting- Cycle days 18-28 and 1-4. Goal is to boost your metabolism through recovery, diet, workout and supplementation strategies.

Buffing- Cycle days 5-18. Goal is to lose weight by employing diet, workout and supplementation strategies.

Cardio- An abbreviated term for cardiovascular training: any activity that raises your heart rate for an amount of time.

Circuit- A type of workout program in which you move from one exercise to the next with little to no rest in between. The goal is to keep your heart rate up the entire workout.

Clean eating- Eating foods high in nutrients and pure from nature. NO refined sugars, processed foods, preservatives, food coloring, etc…

Cycle day (c-day)- The day you are on in your monthly hormonal cycle. The first day of your period is c-day 1.

Cycle length- The number of days between the first day of your period (c-day 1) and the first day of your next period. The average cycle length is 28 days.

Extended Fast- Simply extend the amount of time your body is in fasting. When you sleep, you are in a fasting state. Examples of how to apply this is the dieting rule: "no eating after 8pm" or to utilize fasted cardio.

Fasted Cardio- Cardio activity done first thing in the morning prior to breaking your fast (breakfast). Theoretically it may help burn a higher percentage of fat for fuel.

Hormonal Timing (HT)- The only exercise, diet, mental approach and supplementation lifestyle that incorporates a woman's monthly hormonal cycle.

Hormone-Induced Failure (HIF)- The epidemic women suffer because they do not factor their monthly hormonal cycle into their diet, fitness and supplementation program.

Intervals- A form of cardio exercise in which you alternate between lower and higher intensity levels. They work both the anaerobic and aerobic energy systems. Intervals are considered the most efficient type of cardiovascular training.

Metabolism- The rate at which your body burns calories.

PB- Personal Best

Rally Room (or Team BuffMother Rally Room)- A private internet support group just for women who are members of Team BuffMother. You can find more info about the Rally Room on www.BuffMother.com.

Supplementation- Adding nutrients to your diet in a pill, liquid, or powder form.

Team BuffMother- A group of women that have been inspired by BuffMother! to believe they can live their dreams. Joining is free on www.BuffMother.com.

The Hormonal Timing Pill- the name for our Hormonal Timing supplement system that consist of two formulations the Boosting Pill and a Buffing Pill. They work with a woman's monthly cycle.

The Law of Adaptation- A law stating that our body adapts to the demands we place on it. It is why we can get in shape, and why you may plateau if you don't continually challenge yourself by changing your fitness routine and your diet.

TOM- (Time Of the Month) It is an acronym for your period.

If I can do it…YOU can too!

Seeing is Believing!

Throughout this book you will have a chance to read several great testimonials from my clients. These testimonials are very important because they will enable you to truly BELIEVE in the power of living a Hormonal Timing lifestyle. The visual proof is in the pictures, but the power is revealed through what these women have to say about Hormonal Timing. I have personally been very inspired and motivated by each of these wonderful ladies. It's been so fun to witness their success and I can't wait to witness YOURS!

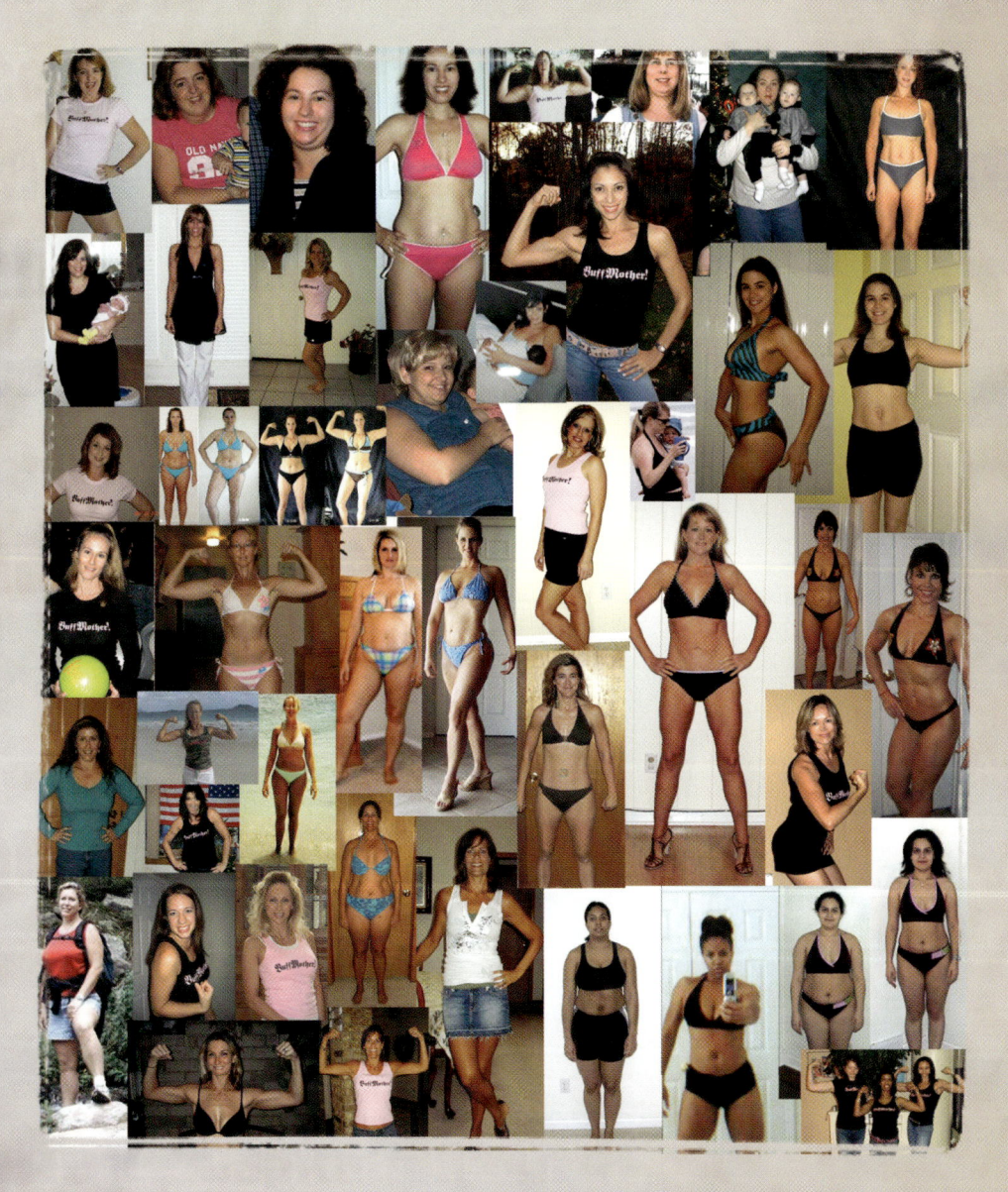

Darcie's Testimony

Darcie Arent is an All-Star!! If I had to pick one characteristic that I admire most it would be her infectious positive energy. She is a very creative person and often shares her creations with us in the Rally Room. Darcie has been applying Hormonal Timing with meticulous effort and has transformed the look of her body from a fluffy mother into that of a young fitness model. Her new body has made her discover that shopping for clothes can be a thrilling experience. During a recent shopping spree Darcie netted 53 new shirts and a boatload of bikini's! I guess that's what happens when everything you try on looks smashing!

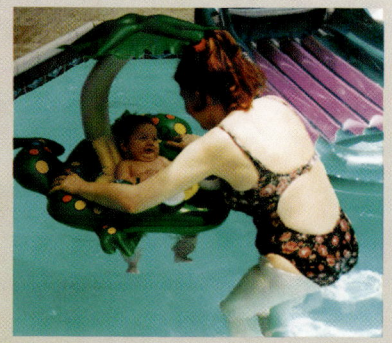

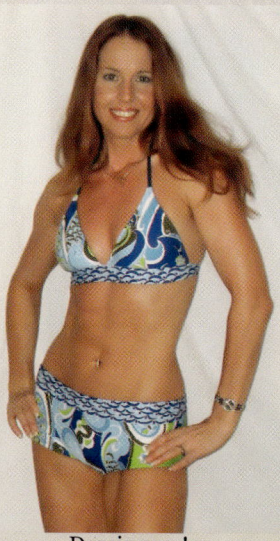

Darcie at her heaviest:

Darcie now!

Can you believe this is the same person?!!!

In her words....

When I got into the rhythm of Hormonal Timing, I could not believe the difference it made to work with my cycle instead of against it. To realize that there are times during the month when I can handle a large workout and times when my body is not equipped to do so was a key moment for me. Knowing that during certain times I need to eat a few more calories took away the guilt of "failure" when I would eat more close to my period. Thanks so much for Hormonal Timing – it has been great!!!– Sept 2006

Update! I have been using the Hormonal Timing system now for 8 months. Not only have I been able to maintain my weight loss but I have added muscle and look even leaner. Pushing myself hard for 2 weeks when my body is able and giving it a break when it needs it has made it easy to stick to my plan. I'm not saying I don't have to work hard – but working with my body has taken away the feeling of struggling against the tide. - May 2007

If I can do it...YOU can too!

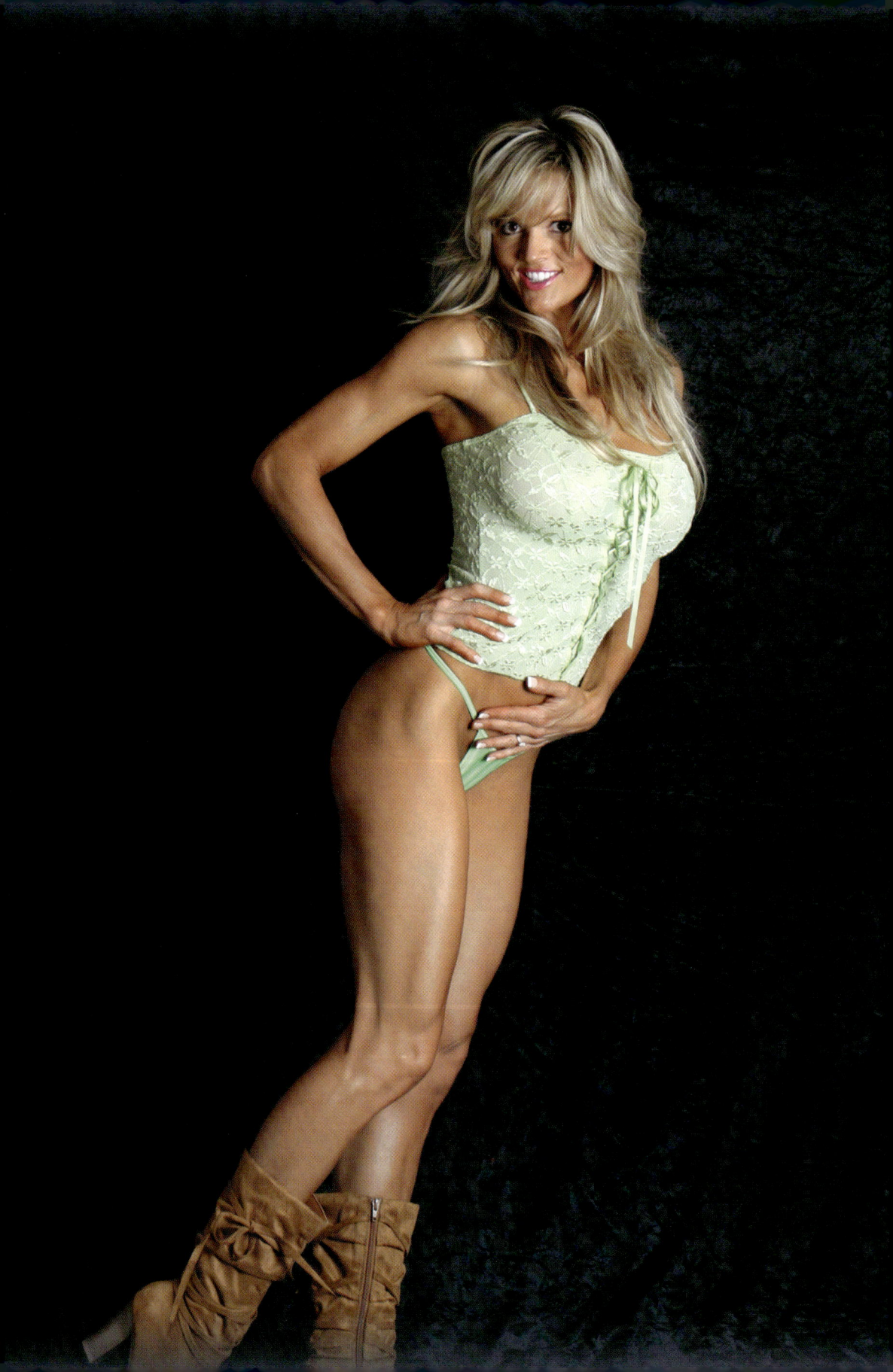

section 2

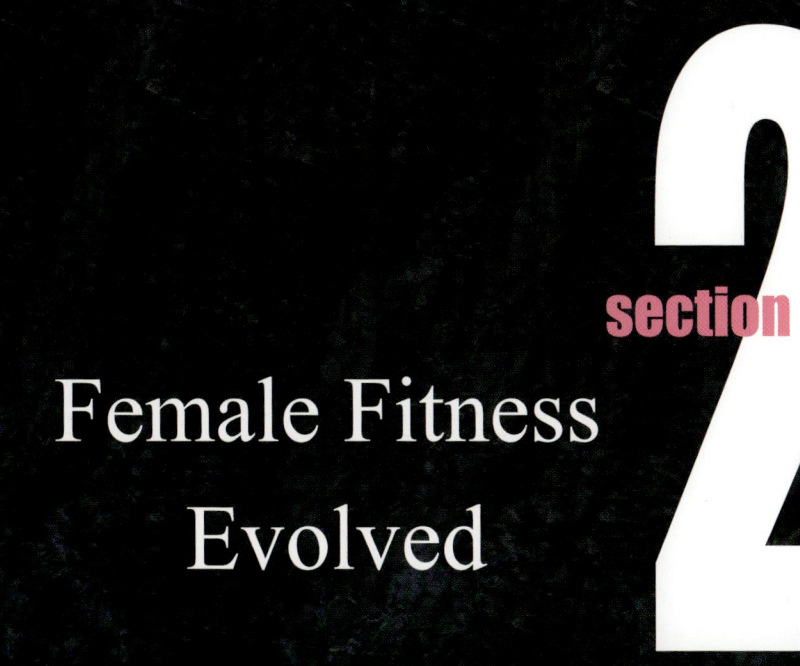

Female Fitness Evolved

Eureka!

You are about to experience a life changing revelation!! I have noticed that every one of my clients has what I call a "light bulb moment" as they learn about Hormonal Timing. This is the moment when you realize that the key to your personal breakthrough rests in the power of your HORMONES! You will know what I mean when it happens. Your life will change forever! Many women feel that they have been battling an invisible enemy, something internal that's preventing them from achieving their vision of success. If you've failed in the past, don't worry. It's not your fault! You were probably just derailed by your hormones. I'll never forget the incredible sense of eureka I felt when it "clicked" for me!

"There have been many great discoveries over time that have completely revolutionized the way we live. The telephone, television, airplanes, computers, cell phones, the internet. . . each of these have transformed virtually every area of our lives! Every discovery happens because someone figures out a different and better way to solve a problem. Hormonal Timing by BuffMother has that kind of "revolutionary" potential." --Dr. Lisa Staudt * see her testimony on the next page.

Unfortunately, there are always conventional mainstream skeptics who don't want to see change. Their favorite word is "impossible." They are very closed minded because they think they know it all, and if there was a better way they would already know about it. This mainstream groupthink attitude is rampant in the women's diet and fitness industry! The goal of mainstream programs is to target the largest market possible so they can earn huge profits. They lump men and women together and don't account for the major differences between us. Most diet and fitness programs are created by marketing people in corporate boardrooms, not by the REAL fitness experts. Nearly all of these programs work better for men than for women. That's right!! Nearly every program ever invented was created by business men for men. Do you want proof? OK, think back to every diet/fitness program you've ever tried or have ever seen advertised. Have any of them ever taken into account your monthly cycle? Do they even mention the fact that your body is completely different on the 5th day of your monthly cycle compared to the 25th day? Never!! I have clients who feel terrible because they fail on program after program just because they are following programs designed for a man. My goal is to scream from the mountain tops:

"DIET AND FITNESS SUCCESS REVOLVES AROUND YOUR HORMONES!!!"

I'm not saying you can't have success on any of these mainstream programs, but if you add Hormonal Timing your results will skyrocket. You will be able to make your body do things that were previously impossible! Hormonal Timing was created for WOMEN ONLY. The Hormonal Timing lifestyle is so incredibly powerful that 5 years from now every mainstream fitness program will be forced to have a Hormonal Timing component. I believe this discovery will completely revolutionize women's fitness.

"Hormonal Timing has been the best kept secret in women's fitness. Once only offered to my private clients for $1200, this powerful information is now in your hands!"

Female Fitness Evolved

Lisa's Testimony

Lisa Staudt knows how to hit it hard and be a success in whatever she does. From the moment I met her through www.BuffMother.com, I have been captivated by her determination to LIVE life to its fullest. She successfully juggled her career as a chiropractor and job as a mother of 3 young children while training hard for her first figure contest. (Which she won!) I know Lisa will accomplish all her goals because she stays positive and always gets it done!

Lisa in Fall 2006

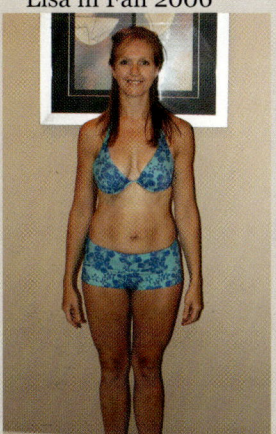

1st Place Winner, Fall '07

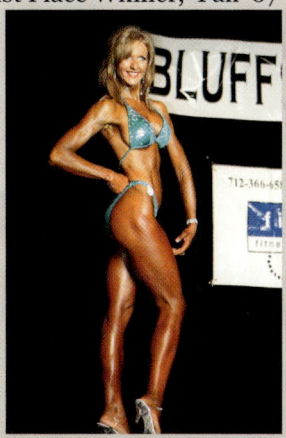

As a chiropractor, Lisa has an amazing view of how Hormonal Timing will change the world of women's fitness:

In her words....

"I think Hormonal Timing (HT) could be a major breakthrough for women's fitness. I love it!! When I first read about it, I thought "this is so cool, it really makes sense." As a chiropractor, I've taken seminars and studied a lot on the female hormones, cycles and nutrition. I think the key point to HT is that your workouts change as you are going through hormonal fluctuations in your cycle. The second half of the month can be a time of stress, increased emotions, depressed feelings, bloating, pain, etc. So having a workout that is less intense and being able to eat more calories just makes sense! Personally Hormonal Timing has helped me establish consistency. The coolest part is that HT is a long term plan, something I will do for life!!"

Are you ready to get started on your own path to success? Let's dive in to the first Foundation....

Female Fitness Evolved

Foundation #1: Realize That You Are in a Battle!

I'm sure you've felt it: that sudden lack of ambition that just seems to overcome you. You might say, "This time I'm going to stick to my plan!" And you do for a while, but then you suddenly realize that you've been slacking for the last 5 days! What happened? You then you blame yourself thinking, "I don't have any self discipline, self control, motivation, etc…" You feel guilty about your lack of willpower.

Maybe you feel like you're close to reaching your goals but just can't quite get there. You work so hard but when you look in the mirror you are always disappointed! You constantly ask yourself, "What am I doing wrong"? What am I missing?!?

The fact is the vast majority of us have a war going on inside. It may be about our diet, exercise habits, smoking, drinking, career issues, relationship problems, etc. Every woman's battle is unique. Sometimes we win and sometimes we lose. We battle against the "visible" enemies of time, obstacles, responsibility, money, and others. However all too often, we are derailed from a victory because of some unknown force. We mysteriously become scattered, lose our energy, feel anxious and fearful, turn negative and doubtful or lose our self-control. An "invisible" enemy comes along and defeats us. It's our HORMONES! Our hormones are the "invisible" enemy, and it's time that we learn how to fight back.

Millions of women fail to reach their diet and fitness goals simply due to their hormones

This affliction is called Hormone-Induced Failure (HIF) and it will sabotage your success unless you're prepared. I believe that <u>HIF</u> is an <u>epidemic</u> in America!

Are you a victim of HIF: Hormone-Induced Failure?

Answer these 5 questions to find out if you have Hormone-Induced Failure:
1. Are you a habitual yo-yo dieter?
2. Do you periodically suffer from uncontrollable cravings that sabotage your efforts to lose weight?
3. Do you start exercise programs and then quit for no apparent reason?
4. Do you ever suffer sudden weight gain that makes you want to quit trying?
5. Do you catch yourself saying things like, "I have no willpower" or "I'm just not motivated…?"

In my experience, most women answer yes to many of the above questions. Most women blame themselves but YOU must understand, IT'S NOT YOUR FAULT!! **Hormone-Induced Failure (HIF) is to blame!!**

Hormones Control Your Diet and Fitness Success!

FACT: Your appetite, cravings, motivation level, mood, energy level, water weight, belly bloat and metabolism are controlled by your hormones!

Hormones control:
Appetite/ junk food cravings
Motivation level/mood
Energy level
Water weight gain/belly bloat
Metabolism
ETC...

Hormones control your appetite (junk food cravings)

Do you have those days when you just wanna eat? I mean really "pig out," on things like doughnuts, cookies, chips, chocolate, etc? It is a sad-but-true fact that our hormones cause us to DESIRE these items. Specifically during the time of the month when your concentrations of hormones are at their highest, you will desire quick easy sources of carbohydrates (carbs), the easiest source being junk food. These carbs spike the secretion of serotonin, your "feel good" hormone so too often you find your cravings seem out of control. What can you do avoid this? Simply, having a plan to eat enough healthy carbs really helps to keep your cravings under control, and supplementing your diet with the proper vitamins and nutrients can help your cravings diminish.

Hormones control your motivation level and mood (mentality)

The psychological effects of hormones are well documented. According to the Mayo Clinic, symptoms of hormone imbalances include feelings of hopelessness, anger, anxiety, low self-esteem, difficulty concentrating, irritability, tension and depression. An imbalance in hormone levels may cause you to feel sad, lonely, apathetic, self-critical, and unsure of yourself. Just a little bit of being "down" can wreak havoc on your diet and fitness efforts.

My motivation to accomplish anything, especially anything hard, often disappears during the second half of my cycle. When I hit day 22 of my cycle, my reason behind working out or dieting gets lost. I say to myself, "Why am I doing this? I don't want to!" I also find myself taking less time out for my other needs. Even simple things like doing my hair, nails, shaving, and putting on make up, become difficult and a pain. Personally, I was never a consistent exerciser until I was aware of my own hormonal lack of motivation, or HIF, and took action against it.

Female Fitness Evolved

On the positive side of things, the instant your hormones drop, signaling your body to menstruate, your motivation will begin to rise again...and after a couple days you will feel powerful and ready to conquer mountains. This powerful feeling typically continues until a few days after ovulation and when you will feel the "lazy bug" hit again. This is when you may fall off your fitness or diet program. Time and time again I have had clients, friends and family who literally "fall off the face of the earth" at this high hormone time of the month. This is classic Hormone Induced Failure (HIF).

Hormones control your energy level and sleep patterns

Do you have days where you are just dragging, limp and lifeless? Yet you can't figure out why? Hormones control your energy levels. Based upon the balance of your hormones in your body your energy levels may be high or low. Each month, energy levels rise and fall according to the balance of estrogen, progesterone and testosterone in your system. If a you are unaware of this cycle when you hit a low energy phase you may think you are just being wimpy, not eating enough, getting sick, etc. BUT, if you know that your low energy is caused by your hormones you will be able to utilize HT to prevent these low-energy days, or at least get through them without beating yourself up about it and losing all momentum. You will be able to honestly tell yourself, I am tired just because of my hormones and tomorrow I will be fine.

As your hormone levels rise toward the end of each month, your sleep may be disturbed, causing energy during the day to be scarce. Often times simply allowing yourself more rest or a nap during this time of the month is all you need to be happier, healthier, and consistent in your fitness efforts. Conversely, after your period is over and through the remainder of the first part of each monthly cycle, your energy levels are high, you sleep deep, and have energy to accomplish your objectives.

Hormones control water weight gain and belly bloat

Oh man! This can be bad!! As a woman, the scale is not your friend for several days of the month. No matter how perfect you may be in your diet and exercise, the scale has a mind of its own when hormones run high. Your rising hormone levels will cause you to retain water toward the end of each monthly cycle. This is part of why you appear "soft" in comparison to a man. Your natural sex hormones help keep your skin full and plump, which is all fine and dandy, until it holds onto 3 pounds more than just the day earlier and fluffs you up so much that your pants don't button! Water retention doesn't just happen in one localized part of your body— it affects your face, hands, feet, belly, butt, etc. Another nasty result of water retention is that our cellulite looks even more dramatic at this time of the month. I point out to my clients that I can actually "see" the hormones in them—it is visible as ripples due to hormone metabolites (toxins), especially in the hips, legs and abdomen. As you become leaner, you will experience greater water weight fluctuations because muscle cells hold a lot more water than fat cells. Don't lose heart when this happens!! It is actually a good sign that you are headed in the right direction with your body composition.

Hormones control your metabolism

As you go through the month, your hormones affect your metabolism (the rate at which your body burns calories). Documented studies show you can actually burn up to an extra 500 calories per day during the week prior to your period. NO WONDER you feel like you want to eat everything in sight! Your body is telling you that you need the extra energy. Why then do you feel horribly guilty if you eat a bit more? Probably because you are already bloated and feel frustrated, so eating extra food seems like the worst thing to do. Don't let guilt turn your fitness quest upside down. Accept that fact that you may need a few more calories right now, plan for that, and enjoy your indulgence. This will enable you to end the cycle of guilty binges and emotional eating before they start.

Hormones control many other aspects that affect your body and life

The list of other ways hormones affect you is long but here are a few: yeast infections, digestive issues, constipation, hair loss, allergies, libido, etc. I've personally been concerned about these symptoms from time to time. Once I connected the symptom to my hormones, I was free from worry because I knew, "It's just my hormones

Every woman is a bit different in regards to her biggest hormonal struggle. But no matter what, there are effects from your hormones--good ones and bad ones--and they must be considered in your diet and fitness program. The key point to know is that there are nutrients, mental strategies, diet, and fitness applications that will help prevent or minimize the bad effects and allow you to capitalize on the good effects. As my program, HT, is applied month after month, you will finally have consistency! Consistency will allow you to realize your full potential and live a fuller, less stressful life.

"Hormones have the power to make you FAT!!
...and the power to make you FIT!!"

Success Tool #1- Identify Your HIF Patterns

The effects of hormones are very sneaky. It is very important that you learn to predict your hormonal patterns. Knowing what to expect is half the battle. For example when striving to prevent Hormone Induced Failure (HIF), if you know that each month on cycle day 25 you suddenly weigh 4 pounds more, you won't get discouraged because you know it's simply your hormones causing water retention. **The key is to know what's coming before it happens by identifying your HIF (Hormone Induced Failure) patterns. The best way to do this is to always <u>chart your cycle</u>.**

Facts about hormonal cycles:
Every woman is unique
- in how hormones affect them
- in their concentrations and ratios of estrogen to progesterone
- in their concentrations and ratios of other key hormones
- in when they ovulate
- in their cycle length
- in their period length, duration and intensity

The below chart shows a <u>generalization</u> of what is happening in your body over the course of your monthly cycle: Cycle day 1(c-day 1) is the first day of your period each month. Ovulation will be roughly mid-cycle (c-day 14) and the average cycle lasts 28 days, but it is not out of the norm to have a slightly shorter or longer cycle. That is why it is important to track each month.

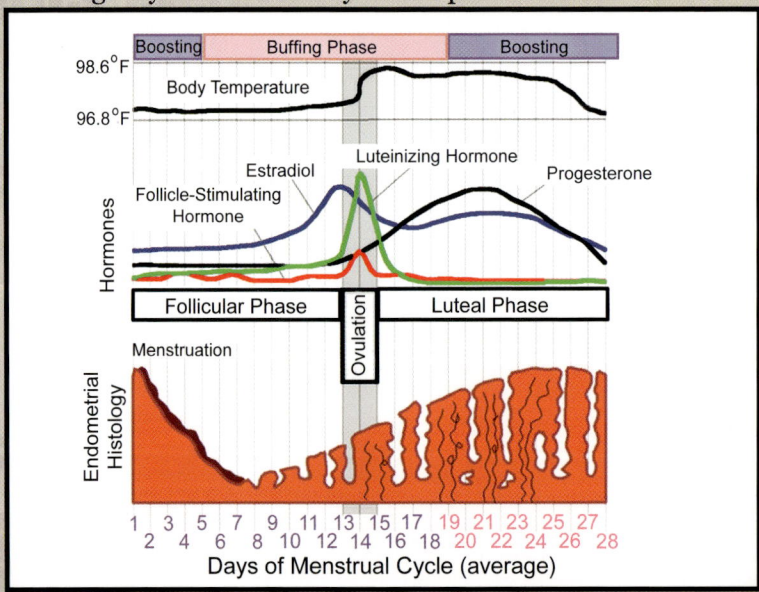

You will have negative mental and physical symptoms:

<u>NOTE Mental symptoms that may be related to your hormones-</u> your motivation level, your mood, your emotions (good or bad), your anger, bad cravings or no appetite, no desire to drink water, lack of mental focus, sexual desire, stress, anxiety, etc... become highly aware of anything that may lead to Hormone-Induced Failure.

<u>NOTE Physical Symptoms that may be associated with hormones-</u>skin breakouts (dry or oily), water weight gain, hunger pangs, upset stomach, no appetite, no desire to drink water, restless sleep, yeast infection, physical pain, weakness, fatigue, bloated, blood flow (heavy days, light days, number of days). Anything that hinders your comfort level, may simply be related to your hormones.

You will have positive symptoms:

Too much of what we hear about hormones is about the negative...but there are also positives caused by our hormones. Often times when things are good we tend to be oblivious. Start paying attention to the good feelings you have both mentally and physically and chart them. Trust me: They are often related to your hormone levels.

Some positive effects related to your hormones:

- Energy
- Zest
- Laughter
- Confidence
- Social
- Outgoing
- Joy
- Peace
- Calm
- Goal oriented
- Sex drive
- Smooth skin
- Good digestion
- Focused
- Motivated
- Mentally strong
- Weight loss
- Strength
- Power
- Quick recovery
- Flexibility
- Build muscle
- Burn Fat
- Good energy stores
- Increased intensity
- Increased drive to win

Once again, you can see hormones affect us in so many ways and that they must be accounted for in your fitness quest!

Female Fitness Evolved

How to chart you hormones daily by using the CHART on the next page

1. **C-day?** Calculate your current cycle day on a normal monthly calendar. The 1st day of your period is c-day 1.

2. **Date?** Note the date and the day of the week (M, T, W, etc..) next to your current c-day (cycle day) on the chart. Start with that day and chart as you move forward.

3. **Weight?** Note your weight each day of the month- take it first thing in the morning for consistency.

4. **Symptoms?** Rate your symptoms. Write "good," "ok" or "bad" below symptoms or make notes similar to the following ideas:
   - **Bloat-** tummy flat? tummy bloat? retaining water?
   - **Mood-** happy or sad? content or frustrated? up or down?
   - **Focus-** motivated, driven, focused, goal-oriented, lazy, scattered?
   - **Stress-** low or high?
   - **Energy-** high or low? tired physically/mentally? sleepy?
   - **Pain-** pain-free or painful? back pain, cramps, joint pain, headache, stiff neck?
   - **Hunger-** no appetite, cravings, hunger pains, unsatisfied?
   - **Strength-** extra weak? extra strong?
   - **Sleep-** good, restless, deep, interrupted (kids), night sweats, bad dreams
   - **Libido-** none, some, responsive, on fire
   - **Others-** yeast infections, oily skin/dry skin, pimples, body odor, etc…

5. **Star-** ★ If you are aware of your ovulation, note that date with a star.

6. **Notes-** Please feel free to write additional notes or chart other symptoms here or in a journal, day planner, blog, etc.

7. **Reference-** Keep each month's chart for you to analyze and refer to later. You will be amazed at the many trends you will identify within just a couple months of charting.

A real life example of how I chart my cycle:

#	C-day Date	Weight	Bloat	Mood	Focus	Stress	Energy	Pain	Hunger	Strength	Sleep	Libido	Other
1	9/19 W	127	BODY	BAD	none	YES	OK	YES	YES	STRONG	bad	NO	
2	9/20 Th	126	tummy	OK	lazy	OK	TIRED!	YES	craving	GOOD	good	NO	moving slow
3	21 F	127	OK	good	OK	OK	TIRED	—	no	OK	good	—	
4	22 Sa	126	GOOD	happy	FOCUSED	OK	GOOD	—	no	weak	deep	OK	
5	23 Su	126	none	happy	goals!		LOTS	good	yes	weak		some	
6	24 M	125	—	good	Driven	BUSY!	↑	sore	yes	weak	Great	YEP	
7	25 T	124	none	—	Zesty	Low	:)	sore	none	better	KIDS	SEXY!	
8	26 W	124	)	—	Great	low	good	—	none	OK	not enough	some	
9	27 Th	124	)	—	NAW	Low	tired	—	none	OK	good	—	
10	28 F	124	flat :)	happy	Good	OK	GOOD	—	none	OK	good	good	
11	29 Sa	124	:)	enemy	YES	HIGH	TONS!	—	none	OK	LOTS!	good	FUN!
12	30 Su	125	water!	good	lazy	OK	OK	—	cravings	OK	OK	horny	
13	10/1 M	125	—	good	FOCUSED	STRESS	tired	BACK	YES	Strong	OK	"	ZITS
14	10/2 T	126	EEK!	happy	NOPE	no	tired	OVARY	none	Strong	bad	OUCH!	BOOBS!
15	3 W	124	good		good	no	LOTS	—	none	weak	OK	GOOD	
16	4 Th	124	:)	so,so	YES	YES	:)	—	none	weak	KIDS	SEXY	
17	5 F	123!	ripped	good	YES	NO	good	Knee	yes-togs	weak	not enough	horny	DATE!
18	6 Sa	123	flat	peace	OK	NO	TIRED	Sore	none	weak	DEEP	good	
19	7 Su	124	good	OK	none	no	TIRED	—	full!	OK	dreams!	nope	stiff
20	8 M	124	good	lonely	lazy	YES	OK	—	hungry	OK	dreams!	OK	
21	9 T	123	good	good	OK	OK	OK	—	very	strong!	deep	lovey	
22	10 W	124	tummy	hermit	OK	YES	OK	—	very	strong	bad	Romance!	
23	11 Th	125	belly	sad	NO	YES	NONE	—	very	strong	OK	"	
24	12 F	126	belly	sad	NO	EEK!	none	—	OK	PB's!!	bad	NO WAY!	
25	13 S	126	belly	OK	good	OK	none	Head	OK	"	bad	"	Yeast
26	14 Su	128	BODY	OK	low	low	OK	head	Starving	"	sweats	OK	fight!
27	15 M	128	BODY	Crabby	OK	high	low	back	cravings	"	sweats	horny	
28	16 T	126	better	MAD	NONE	YES	good	back	"	weaker	sweats	OK	allergies

pink days = Buffing Phase
purple days = Boosting Phase

Female Fitness Evolved
29

Predicting Numerous Patterns

You will see patterns monthly and be able to identify when your "toughest" days occur. You may see things that you never considered related to your hormones become apparently connected as you chart. Have you ever considered allergies or getting a cold as being related to hormones? What about being accident prone? As you progress in your hormonal timing you will realize all sorts of interesting correlations. The most important factor in charting is self awareness, recognizing your hormonal fluctuations and then working with your body versus fighting it. There are certain days when you should just rest instead of pushing hard. You may also realize there are days when you just won't feel like working out, but because you know if you do it you will feel better and have the stress relief you desperately need, you will just have to do it anyway. A great thing that I've been able to do with many of my clients is that as we learn about their own HIF, we'll customize their own Buffing and Boosting plans according to their individual cycle.

Some answers to "Why should I chart?":

Weight- Chart your weight daily so you don't FREAK out when your hormones cause you to retain water. Ovulation will cause a bit of water retention, be prepared for it. If you know that last month you gained 3 pounds on day 14 of your cycle and that all those pounds were gone by day 16 you will be able to reason yourself out of a tizzy. Also, if you know that on day 25, 26 and 27 you gained 2 pounds each day, but by day 3 of your next cycle all 6 of those pounds were gone, you will be able to almost ignore those pounds. Charting your cycle will allow you to know your "REAL" weight versus a hormone induced "high" weight or a dehydrated extra "low" weight. In one week, my weight can easily fluctuate up to 7 pounds! I can go from a bit dehydrated 123 to a bloated 130 in a matter of days! But, I have been charting and I know that my REAL weight is about 126. I now understand how, why, when and for how long fluctuations occur.

Libido- Your libido (sex drive) is closely related to your hormonal cycle. As you track it, you will see patterns and realize when you are most sexually responsive, when you feel you least sexual and when you have the most sexual confidence. Knowing this information and sharing it with your husband/partner will increase the sexual happiness in your relationship. See more about this in the Bonus Section: Hormonal Timing SEX!

If you have ovaries you have a hormonal cycle

If you are on "the pill" or any other form of prescribed "hormone therapy" (patch, depo, estrogen cream, progesterone cream, etc) you will still have a natural cycle of hormones...make sure to chart your symptoms. The added benefit of knowing how your body responds to that particular type of birth control may come in handy at your next doctor visit. If you take the pill, I would recommend opting to take the traditional 28 day cycle of pills which contain a week of "inactive" placebo pills to allow for monthly bleeding (your period). Also if you have the option of being "natural" go for it, I feel it is most often the optimal choice.

In the case of a hysterectomy, if you still have your ovaries, you still have a monthly hormone cycle. Likewise, if you are going through menopause or you're post-menopausal you still have a cycle ....make sure to chart. Don't assume that if you don't bleed monthly you are not having cyclical hormone fluctuations. You do! Without a period you won't know what cycle day you are on in your month, so simply use a calendar to chart your symptoms. Soon you will clearly see the cycle of your hormones from low to high.

Summary of Section II:

- Many women feel that they have been battling an invisible enemy, something internal that's preventing them from achieving their vision of success.
- Until now, MEN have ruled the fitness world and ignored the fact that women's bodies have a hormonal cycle.
- Eureka!! Ladies, your diet and fitness success must revolve around your HORMONES.

Foundation #1- Recognize That You Are In a Battle; you are under ATTACK by an invisible enemy! Hormone Induced-Failure is a real epidemic. You must consider how your hormones affect you so you have a chance to win the WAR.

Hormones control every critical area pertaining to your diet and fitness success!

Appetite/ Junk food cravings
Motivation level/Mood
Energy level
Water weight gain
Metabolism
ETC...

Success Tool #1- Identify Your HIF Patterns, by tracking your cycle.

KNOWLEDGE IS POWER!

Female Fitness Evolved

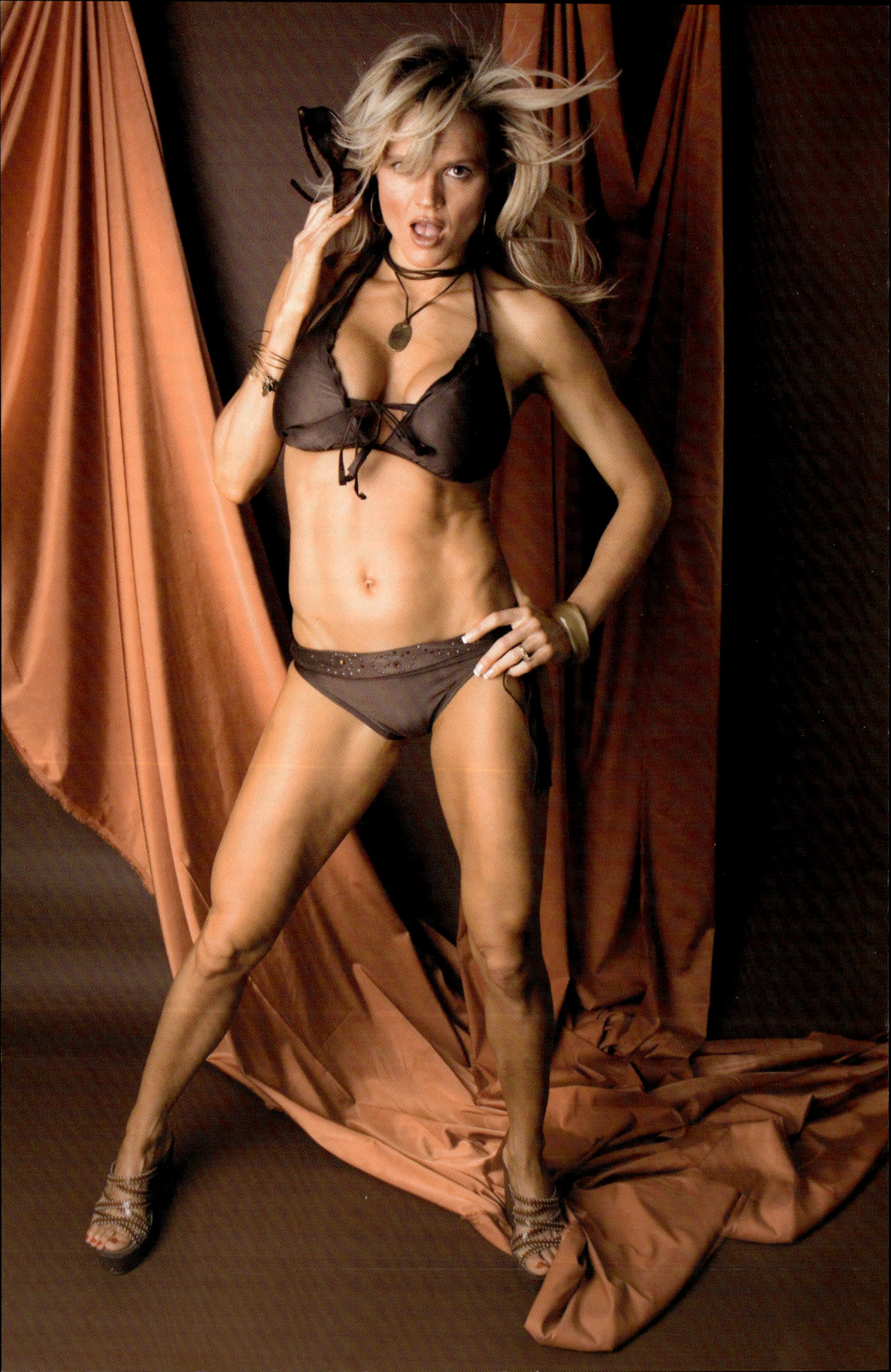

section 3

Harness the POWER of your Hormones!

Foundation #2: Hormonal Timing™

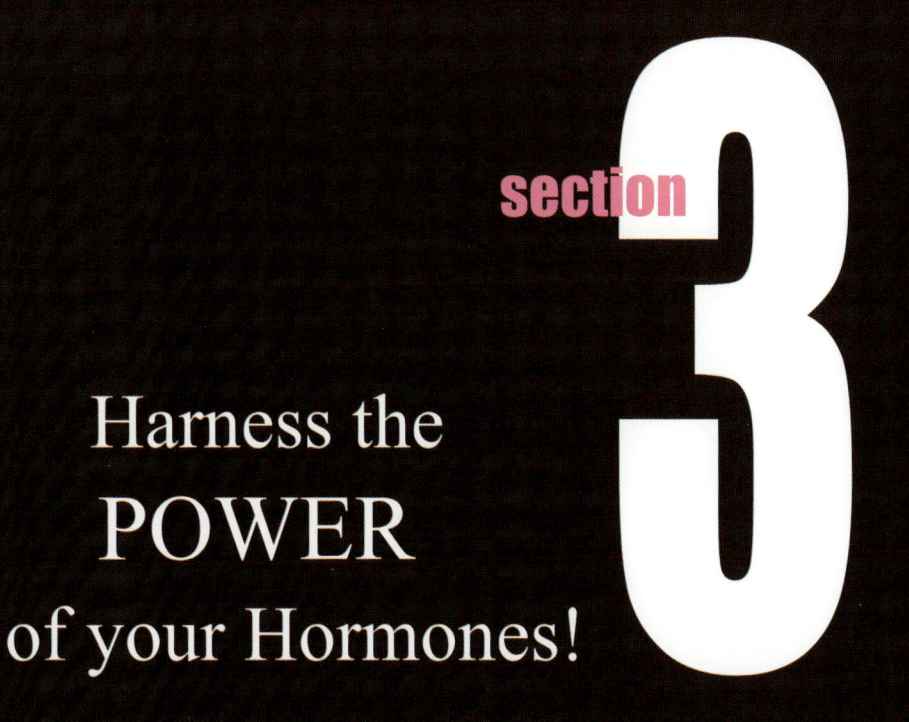

What is Hormonal Timing™? Simply put, it is the CURE to Hormone-Induced Failure! Hormonal Timing's secret is that you will **work with** your body and your hormones allowing you to STOP being at war with yourself! Once you embrace your hormones and allow them to work for you, you will be happier, healthier and in better shape than ever! Hormonal Timing will teach you how to capitalize on the good effects of your hormones and negate the bad effects. This will allow you to build incredible momentum to break through previous limitations. Hormonal Timing will allow you to finally achieve your fitness and diet goals!!

The BASICS of how Hormonal Timing™ works:

- You have two distinct phases of your monthly cycle: the first half (good time) and the second half (when Hormone-Induced Failure typically strikes). Each phase is an average 2 weeks in duration.
- Hormonal Timing synchronizes your workout, diet and supplement routine with these 2 distinct environments. The first phase is called Buffing and the second is Boosting. Your workouts, diet and supplement prescription are distinct during the two phases.
- Optimal hormonal conditions are capitalized on during each of the phases to burn fat and transform your body.
- As you get in sync with your body through using Hormonal Timing, you will be able to overcome the mental and physical obstacles that have sabotaged your success in the past. You will overcome HIF!
- Hormonal Timing can work with any exercise and diet program! If you love your current diet and your workouts, by simply applying a few Hormonal Timing adaptations your results will be magnified!
- The Hormonal Timing Pill (supplement system) helps restore the natural balance of nutrients that support the production of hormones in your body and ultimately helps to minimize or eliminate an imbalance of hormones that cause HIF.
- The two pill formulations (Buffing and Boosting) are specific to the environment present in your body during that hormonal phase and will optimize your body's response to the prescribed exercise and diet of that phase. They will nourish your body to help negate the bad effects and optimize the good effects during both the Buffing and Boosting phase.

The bottom line: Your hormones have the power to make you fat and your hormones have the power to make you thin!!

Harness the power of your hormones to unlock the body inside your body; **IT IS Beautiful!!**

Dr. Testimonials

The following two testimonials are from medical doctors who enrolled in my 8-week training program called the "Miracle 8." I walked them through an 8-week, hands-on Hormonal Timing training program. It involved daily e-mails, twice weekly phone calls and continual adjustment of their program based on their progress and needs. They learned all the information in this book over those 8 weeks and were given the wisdom they needed to succeed on Hormonal Timing for a life time.

In her words....

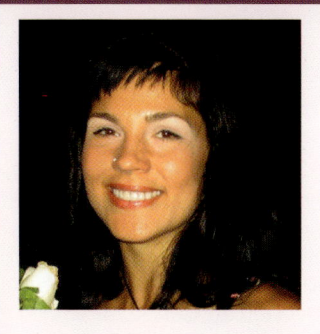

Testimony of Dr. Angela Franko, MD

Michelle Berger's theory of Hormonal Timing provides a remarkable and extremely effective approach to achieving a leaner, more muscular physique. It can benefit any woman who is interested in changing her body shape, losing unwanted fat, or simply trying to improve her overall fitness levels. Her concept specifically caters to the female population because unlike other programs out there, it utilizes a woman's natural hormonal milieu as dictated by her monthly cycles. This strategy, in combination with appropriate nutrition and training sets the stage for a powerful bodily response toward desired fitness goals.

Personally I have tried many programs in the past and while I have achieved results, there comes a point when the results are limited and I fall short of meeting my goals. Like many other frustrated women, I felt like I was working against myself, almost as if something was holding me back despite doing everything "correctly", or so I thought. Michelle's concept particularly intrigued me, as never before had I heard of synchronizing training and nutrition with one's monthly cycle. The simple fact that Michelle, a mother of four can look as amazingly fit as she does, shows that she is onto something unique.

The benefits of Hormonal Timing are numerous. For one, there is a huge metabolic advantage to coordinate one's hormonal fluctuations with modifications in diet and training. During the first ("follicular") phase of the month, the body is more primed for catabolism, so the focus lies in shedding fat during this period. The hormonal state of latter ("luteal") phase enhances anabolic processes, so this time period is ideal for adding muscle. Altering the diet and training components with the two phases of the monthly cycle can achieve marked body transformation. This means you see big results and you see them faster. For me, I could literally watch my progress by means of my body measurements and photographs: it was clear that I was dropping fat and adding muscle. Another advantage to Michelle's system is that it helps one to circumvent adaptation. By varying the elements of nutrition, cardio and resistance training with the "Buffing" and "Boosting" phases, it keeps the body guessing. The metabolism stays revved and in the end, progress is made while avoiding stagnation. In my opinion, one of the most significant benefits to Hormonal Timing is that it truly helps from a psychological viewpoint. Monthly hormonal changes can greatly alter mood and energy levels, which can make it difficult to stay motivated to train and eat properly. To be more aware of ones menstrual cycle helps to understand the basis for those feelings of fatigue, sluggishness and irritability that many women experience prior to their period. To appreciate that this trying time is short lived, it becomes easier to persist through it and remain focused on the desired goal. Last but not least, another key element to Michelle's program is her recommended use of supplements. For instance, the use of vitamin B6, magnesium, chromium and calcium helps to minimize premenstrual symptoms (PMS), such as added water weight, irritability and intensified sugar cravings. Another beneficial supplement, l-glutamine helps to enhance muscle recovery so that effective training sessions can resume without excessive soreness.

Overall, I highly recommend Michelle's program of Hormonal Timing to any woman who wants to improve her physique and/or fitness levels. Due to the positive changes I have personally experienced in using her program, she undoubtedly has my continued support. This valuable program would be an asset to any woman who has the aspiration to achieve a fit and healthy lifestyle.

-Angela Franko, MD   Calgary, Alberta, CANADA

Harness the Power of your Hormones

In her words....

Testimony of Dr. Carol Sonatore, MD

Working with Michelle as my online trainer has been a great experience. I specifically chose to work with her because of the marked changes in her own body composition that she achieved, and her background in exercise physiology. It was important to me as a woman to work with another female who I admire. And it was important as a physician to work with someone I felt was very knowledgeable. Prior to my experience with Michelle, when I wanted to lose weight, I would focus on drastically reducing my caloric intake, and if I exercised more, it would be by adding more aerobic type exercise to my routine. As a doctor, I know theoretically that increasing muscle mass will cause more calories to be burned 24 hours a day. However, like many women, I was afraid of becoming too "big" especially in my hips and thighs, where I carry most of my weight. My program, devised by Michelle, focused on weight training and building muscle. The aerobic training was focused on interval training of approximately only 20 minutes duration. We had many discussions during the 8 weeks, including how muscle becomes more "dense" with training, as the fat marbled within the muscle is being burned away. This was one of the many revelations I learned, and it helped to alleviate my fears about becoming "big."

In addition to the exercise program, I was impressed with Michelle's recommended diet and supplementation regimen. Of particular interest was her theory of Hormonal Timing. For instance, during ovulation or the later part of the menstrual cycle, Michelle had suggested extra carbohydrate intake, as well as a heavier lifting routine. This worked very well with my increased cravings, and felt like a natural adjustment to the workout and diet. She referred that as the "Boosting phase" of the cycle. During the "Buffing phase," during/after menstruation, focus was on adding some more cardio, and circuit type weight training – keeping an elevated heart rate. Overall, this idea of adjusting your eating and exercise program to your body's needs was unique, yet felt very natural. Not only did it produce results, it made her program easy to stick with.

I made sure to take the supplements that Michelle suggested. Being a doctor and also having a nutrition background, I am able to recognize unsafe supplementation, and none of Michelle's suggestions came close to that. She happens to be a very bright as well as responsible person! From a dietary standpoint, I also minimized dairy consumption, increased my water intake and ate to fuel my workouts, as suggested by Michelle. I used protein supplementation as well to make it easier to get in the suggested amount of protein per day. My results were wonderful! Aside from losing inches and fat, I noticed other changes: The acne on my chest cleared up, and I became markedly more energetic. My face was less puffy, and I had less noticeable circles under my eyes as well.

I highly recommend Michelle as an online trainer and health coach. Her unique program incorporating Hormonal Timing with your workout, supplementation and diet recommendations have helped me to achieve better health, vitality and lose the fat!

-Carol Sonatore, MD
New Jersey

How To Harness The Power of Your Hormones

Hormonal Timing employs 3 simple strategies that allow you to harness the power of your hormones so that you can experience radical changes in your body as well as your mind!

1. **Education-** Knowledge is power! I will show you what to do, when to do it and most importantly why you need to do it. You must have a plan in place that capitalizes on the good effects and negates the bad effects of your hormones. If you aren't working with your hormones, you are working against them! As you learned in "Success Tool #1," knowing when and what to expect from your hormone fluctuations is a key to success.

2. **Diet/Fitness-** We will coordinate your diet and fitness program with what your body naturally wants to do. You will respond best to different things at different times depending on your hormonal cycle. Here's a good comparison: If you were to try and get pregnant at the wrong time of the month, you will have a rough time. The same holds true with diet and fitness. Your cycle will determine what works at any given time during the month. We are not meant to fight our bodies. We need to embrace what makes women different than men and utilize those differences to our advantage. Realize that there are ton of GREAT benefits to having a hormonal cycle. We can use those benefits to completely revolutionize your body. Simply "planning" to include your body's cycle into your diet and fitness program creates a coordinated synergy that eliminates frustration and creates to success.

3. **Supplementation-** As your hormones fluctuate throughout the month, your nutritional needs fluctuate also. It is critical that your supplementation is adjusted to account for these fluctuations. I believe much of the credit for my success belongs to the completely revolutionary Hormonal Timing Pill. The Buffing and Boosting formulations were made to nourish your body on a cellular level according to your monthly cycle. We experimented for years to get the formulation right and I know they will make a big difference in your life. The Hormonal Timing Pill will help you gain momentum as your body transitions through the 2 main hormonal environments of each month. The longer you maintain proper supplementation, your body will function optimally, and the more dramatic your results will become.

"Hormonal Timing changes everything!! You are a woman. Take advantage of it!"

Now let's take a deeper look at the 2 main hormonal environments which exist in your body throughout your monthly cycle. I have termed them the "Buffing" phase and the "Boosting" phase. These two phases work together towards rebuilding your body. Enabling you to operate with increased consistency that will generate the momentum you need to reach your potential.

Success Tool #2- Buffing and Boosting

Buffing- Cycle days 5-18

The main goal of Buffing is to go all out in every area of your life! This is the time to really push your workouts and FOCUS on keeping your diet as "perfect" as possible! Buffing only lasts for 2 weeks so I really want you to step it up during this phase. You can do anything for just 2 weeks, right? You will make huge progress during Buffing! Here's why:

During cycle days 5-18
- Hormonally, your body is "set up" for successful weight loss.
- Your body "feels good," works efficiently and effectively.
- Your body responds well to diet change and intense workouts.
- Your mind is clearer.
- You generally feel positive about life.
- You have more focus and drive to accomplish your goals.

Let's capitalize on the good effects of the low hormonal levels in your system by utilizing the....

Buffing: Keys to Success

#1 Mental Focus

Mentally you are on and ready to ATTAIN GOALS during Buffing

When was the last time you had an inner drive to set and accomplish new goals? Do you know what cycle day you were on? I bet it was during the Buffing phase of your month. During or just after your period until after ovulation you will be typically much happier, focused, more driven, positive, energized, determined, and courageous. During Buffing you typically DO what you PLAN to do which is so gratifying and creates huge momentum. Knowing that your hormone levels are contributing to this zest will allow you to capitalize even more on this "happy time" of the month. Hormonal Timing takes this into account. It is very smart to push yourself and plan to be aggressive in your fitness and diet during Buffing. Your body will respond amazingly well and you should expect to see results in every measure of success. Go ahead and apply this concept into all areas of your life. During Buffing: Set new goals for your relationships, finances, work life, spiritual life, your family, etc. You will be amazed at how much you can accomplish in just 2 weeks!

#2 Nutrition and Diet Goals

GOAL = Lose weight! during Buffing

As cycle day 5 approaches you need to ask yourself, "How much weight can I lose during the next 2 weeks?" You need to have complete focus on losing as much weight as possible during these 2 weeks of the month. Attack it from all angles, but do it the smart, healthy way. The great news is your body wants to lose weight! You have lower levels of hormones in your system during this portion of the month. As a result, your body is in a weight loss mode. It is also very responsive to diet and exercise which magnifies positive results even further. You have every reason to really go for it during Buffing. The scale is your friend and life is good! AWARENESS is the KEY! Now that you know the physical environment that exists during this time of the month, you can really capitalize on it with maximum effort.

Eat clean nutritious foods

Focus on eating CLEAN during this 2 week phase! Give 100 percent effort toward losing weight. You need to take time every day to plan your attack in order to attain your desired results. You need to have a couple more servings of green veggies and lower your complex carbohydrate intake to the minimum needed to support your workouts. Since your calories will be on the low end, you want the most nutrient-dense foods. Before you eat something think "what good is this food going to do for my body?" If you can't come up with a good answer, don't eat it! Please refer the Diet section on page 100 for some great ideas on CLEAN foods.

I try harder than ever to refrain from "cheating" during Buffing. HT allows you to cheat a little in just 2 short weeks but not now. Your weight loss won't be without effort and sacrifice, but you can do anything for 2 weeks, right? Keep your focus on doing your best during these 2 weeks because you know that you will be rewarded with SPECTACULAR results. You can be comforted in knowing you will get a "break" when you hit your Boosting phase.

Remember: To lose weight you need a caloric deficit

Your body needs a caloric deficit to lose weight. You need to be at roughly a 300-500 calorie deficit per day in order to lose weight. However, you also need to have enough calories to support your workouts, lifestyle and overall health. Be aware that Buffing is not a license to starve yourself—you still need to keep your protein levels high and focus on eating only nutrient-dense foods. You also need to make sure to keep fueling your workouts properly. You will not have good workouts if you are trying to exercise with no fuel.   Please refer to chapter 5 for diet specifics. Constantly reinforce the importance of NUTRIFYING your body. Remember you are in this for the long-term, to create a legacy of HEALTH. Not an unattainable lifestyle of starvation.

Make sure to take The Hormonal Timing Pill (Pink Buffing Pill)!! It will support your efforts! We formulated the Buffing Pill to guard your body from breaking down during this phase. I don't want you to lose muscle mass and I don't want you to get sick from a reduced immune function.

#3 Workouts

Workouts: Work with your POSITIVE MENTAL ATTITUDE (PMA) during Buffing.

Most women naturally experience a much more positive outlook and have more mental strength and determination between c-days 5-18 (Buffing). Let's put to use the GREAT positive attitude, mental strength and determination you have during Buffing. Mentally it is "just easier" to do intense workouts and "activity" during Buffing. Intense determination and a "no excuses" attitude characterize how you feel about physically conquering our workouts during Buffing. Take advantage of your SPUNK and up the frequency of your cardio/interval workouts. Also, since you may have more confidence and courage at this time of the month this is a good time to join a new gym or try a new, different workout routine or class. No matter what activity you choose to do, do all you can for 2 weeks to lose fat, be relentless in your workouts, hit them hard, be focused and intense!

Body Buffing- Move it to lose it

When you buff your nails to get them looking great, it takes a lot of movement and perfecting type moves. Get the same attitude towards your body. In your weight lifting you can go for more fat loss by using circuit style training, taking less rest time between exercises or have an "active rest time" between sets by doing ab work, jumping rope, or another activity that keeps your heart rate up. This extra focus on exercise during Buffing will aid in fat burning and increase your caloric deficit.

Since your body needs less fuel to operate at this time of the month, doing 20 minutes of cardio immediately in the morning prior to breakfast (fasted cardio) may increase fat utilization as your body's fuel. Also, enforcing a general rule like no eating after 7pm will help you keep your calories in check and extend your fast so that your body has more of a chance to burn its stored fat for fuel. Keep in mind that Buffing is just for 2 weeks! The only time I utilize doing some cardio in a fasted state and/or extending my fast is during the Buffing phase.

#4 Cycle Awareness Tidbit - Buffing

Another item of interest during Buffing, is that during the second week of the month you will typically ovulate. This is a mini HIGH hormone time for you, which may cause 1-2 days of lackluster performance, cravings and possible water weight gain. Be staunch through this time in your workouts and diet. You will have 3-4 more days after ovulation to see good Buffing results before you start Boosting.

Summary of Buffing- Cycle Days 5-18:

1. Mental Focus- Your goal is to lose weight through exercise and diet. Set goals- use the strong mental focus to accomplish weight loss. Your lower hormone levels allow your body to release weight and toxins.
2. Nutrition and Diet- Consume a negative caloric intake (-500 cals). Your appetite should be manageable and easily controlled. Strive to eat perfect, plan to sacrifice for results, and take The Hormonal Timing Pill which is formulated to support your hormonal environment and weight loss goals.
3. Workouts- Prescribed exercise is more intense, frequent, and weight loss driven. Buffing exercise aids in weight loss by promoting fat burning and increases your caloric deficit.
4. Cycle Awareness Tidbit- Beware of Ovulation, it can be similar to a mini PMS.

Buffing Reminder Chart

Be relentless- give it 110%
Think, "I can do anything for 2 weeks!"
Focus on weight loss and diet- caloric deficit
Eat CLEAN to lose weight
Do extra activities and cardio
Buff your body- BODY Buffing
Be aware of your Ovulation
Take The Hormonal Timing Pill (pink) Buffing Pill daily

"Hormones are the problem but they are also the solution!"

Boosting- C-day 19-28 and 1-4

Boosting- "the second half of the month"- HIF most often strikes during these two weeks. Keep your mindset determined to BELIEVE! Tell yourself over and over you can reach your goals, and any negative thought or feeling must be combated with: "It is just my hormones!! They are trying to keep me fat!"

Mentally keep an "It's just my hormones" mindset when:
- When the scale suddenly shoots up a few pounds.
- When you don't feel like working out.
- When you feel sad, alone and emotional.
- When you wonder "why am I doing this?"
- When you may feel totally lazy and uninspired.
- When you feel like a failure.
- When you feel guilt creeping in.
- When you feel down and like all effort is in vain.
- When your body seems unresponsive to your diet and workout efforts.
- When your body feels fluffy and your cellulite looks worse than ever.

YOUR rebuttal to all of these feelings, thoughts and events needs to be:
"It's *just* my hormones"!

Let's learn to capitalize on the "good" effects of extra hormones in your system and head off the bad effects by utilizing the....

Boosting Keys to Success

#1 Mental Focus

Take A BREAK during Boosting

Boosting is a MENTAL break from the "perfect" diet and intense workout routine—you may need to take an extra day off to relax, repair and recover each week. That's okay! You may need to have a few more treats. That's okay! Think of Hormonal Timing as a long-term solution. In the long term, we all need to be able to live, laugh and love life!! SO let's plan these times into our diet and fitness routine during the time of the month when our bodies naturally want and need to relax more.

However, the Boosting phase is not a license to throw all good diet and fitness habits out the window. You will not be able to move forward overall if each time Boosting rolls around you go completely backwards. Your goal is to maintain where you are at, so you still need to keep tabs on yourself. You need to be disciplined by keeping your caloric intakes at a reasonable maintenance level and keep up with the workouts you plan. The 5-4-3-2-1 diet that I will detail later on will allow you to have freedom in your food choices and easily maintain your diet progress. Stay focused on maintenance- try to keep the scale steady!! By staying focused on maintenance you will maintain momentum. For instance, plan to workout 4 days a week during Boosting vs. the 5 days you worked out during Buffing. Or cut your workout duration; just doing something will keep your momentum moving in the right direction. You will also need to keep your "why" in the forefront of your thoughts and utilize all the Success Tools in this book to keep your brain "in shape" and energy high. Read more on this in the next section titled "Train Your Brain" starting on page 50.

#2 Nutrition and Diet Goals

Give your "diet" a BOOST during Boosting

When you hear someone say, "my metabolism is shot," they are typically referring to the fact that their body doesn't burn as many calories as they'd like it to on a daily basis. If you are constantly living on a very low caloric intake your body will adjust and become more efficient with its energy usage causing your metabolism to slow down. Studies have shown that in just 2 weeks our body adjusts and adapts to its caloric intake and activity level. This is called The Law of Adaptation which is the fact that your body gets used to how you treat it and adapts. Take this specific example; If you only fed your body 1000 calories a day, soon your body will do all it can to slow its metabolism in order to only utilize 1000 calories a day. On the other hand, if you feed your body 2500 calories a day, your body will adjust and learn to expect that many calories a day thus raising your metabolic rate in order to at least try to use all of those calories each day. This adaptation leads to plateaus in diet progress and is why your body needs a break from low calorie dieting.

Your metabolism will thank you if you take a step away from "diet food" during Boosting focus on eating more normal foods within a specific portion size. Don't go overboard, but incorporate an extra serving of good food daily, and allow yourself a treat. You need a few extra calories and a little reprieve from "HARD dieting" to prevent a progressively slower metabolism resulting in a physical plateau and a mental burn out. Take comfort in knowing that eating a bit more during Boosting is actually helping you by BOOSTING your metabolism. You will be healthier and more successful in the long-term. As you stick to your plan of maintenance, any extra weight you experience is just water and an increase in glucose (energy) stores. Please be aware that even if you are eating perfect, you may gain a bit of water weight. That weight will come off as soon as your cycle is over! It is just your hormones! They cause you to retain water weight. Make sure to chart this info so that you can be aware for the next month and prepared to deal with it—knowledge is powerful!!

#3 Workouts

Less intense focus on your workouts during Boosting
Allow yourself a bit less intensity and a bit more relaxation during your workouts and in your life overall. You may want to schedule yourself an extra day off during this time of your cycle, since you may find it hard to keep the pace you enjoyed during Buffing. The extra rest will help you recoup physically and mentally for your next Buffing phase. Also mentally it may be easier to lift than to do cardio during this phase, so up the frequency of your lifting workouts (or vise versa, if you like cardio better). Do what you enjoy most for your workouts. Just maintain positive momentum and make an effort to focus on doing something. Something is way better than nothing. You need the stress relief and momentum more than ever!

Capitalize on the opportunity of having EXTRA hormones in your body.
During Boosting, your body is set to rest, recover, repair, rebuild. This is part of why we have such trouble controlling our diets during PMS--our body is preparing for possible pregnancy and wants to build the best environment possible. You have more hormones in your system and you can use those hormones to build some fat-burning muscles and boost your metabolism. When you place more emphasis on strength training moves and get aggressive toward challenging your muscles during your Boosting workouts, your body will respond by building muscle. I have clients amazed by how strong they are during the Boosting portion of their cycle. That combined with the little extra food and rest you get during this time of the month, you can boost your metabolism and transform your body into a literal FAT FURNACE!

This is a great time of the month to implement a more advanced strength training program or hook up with a trainer to learn some new lifting exercises...think about rebuilding your body into its former glory. Can you remember those days when you could eat whatever you'd like and not gain a pound? That's the power of muscle and a boosted metabolism. Let's reverse the clock and rebuild that youthful muscle and powerful metabolism.

Advantages to working out through your hormones during Boosting:
1. Stress relief is the biggest one. Release of endorphins from exercise is needed.
2. Sweating will eliminate extra water weight.
3. Your lymphatic system is activated by muscle movement, so exercise will allow your body to release toxins. You need to move in order to "squeeze" the fat and toxins out of your body.
4. The extra hormones in your body give you more muscle building ability so strength training is extra productive and effective.

5. FAT BURNING is increased. Research shows that your body chooses fat for fuel at a higher rate at this time of the month. If you can force yourself to get in some good workouts, they will be very effective.

#4 Cycle Awareness Tidbit - Boosting

Another interesting finding about hormones is that during the week prior to their period women can burn up to 500 calories more each day. No wonder we are so hungry during that time of the month! So know that if you can just make it through to the "other side," to your Buffing phase, without getting out of control, you will see the fruits of your labor!

Summary of Boosting- Cycle Days 19-28 and 1-4

1. Mental Focus: Goal is to maintain weight and boost metabolism. Hormone levels rise creating a greater occurrence of HIF.
2. Nutrition and Diet goals - consume maintenance level calories. Take The Hormonal Timing Pill (purple Boosting pill) which is formulated to help negate the hormonal symptoms prevalent during this phase.
3. Workouts: Exercise is less intense. Focused on Boosting metabolism and regaining youthful muscle. Try to get more rest and recover in preparation for your next Buffing phase.
4. Cycle Awareness Tidbit: It's okay to eat a little more. Your body burns up to 500 more calories per day the week before period.

Boosting Reminder Chart

Rest a bit more- slow the pace
Realize, "It's just my hormones"
Boost your metabolism- eat to fuel your workouts
Maintain your weight loss
Cut back on workout frequency or duration
Focus on doing "something"; strength training is extra productive
You're hungrier because you need more food
Take The Hormonal Timing Pill (purple) Boosting Pill daily

"Women will get in sync with their bodies and be able to overcome the mental and physical obstacles that sabotaged their success in the past."

Harness the Power of your Hormones

How Buffing and Boosting Work Together...to build your body into a healthy fat burning machine:

- Alternating Buffing and Boosting gives you consistency and momentum that is easy to maintain over time. The two week phases are long enough to focus and long enough for results. You will be mentally and physically "pumped up" for each phase as it approaches.

- As you progress through the phases of Buffing and Boosting, you will use the Law of Adaptation to your advantage. After a boosting phase, your metabolism is cranked up from your consumption of more calories. The quick cut in calories once you start Buffing causes your body to respond immediately with weight loss.

- Buffing and Boosting capitalize on the hormonal environment present in your body and allows you to work in harmony with it. The plan enables you to lose weight when your body is poised to do so, and regain youthful muscle in the same regard.

- The Boosting phase of Hormonal Timing prevents physical and mental burn out because it is a built-in rest period.

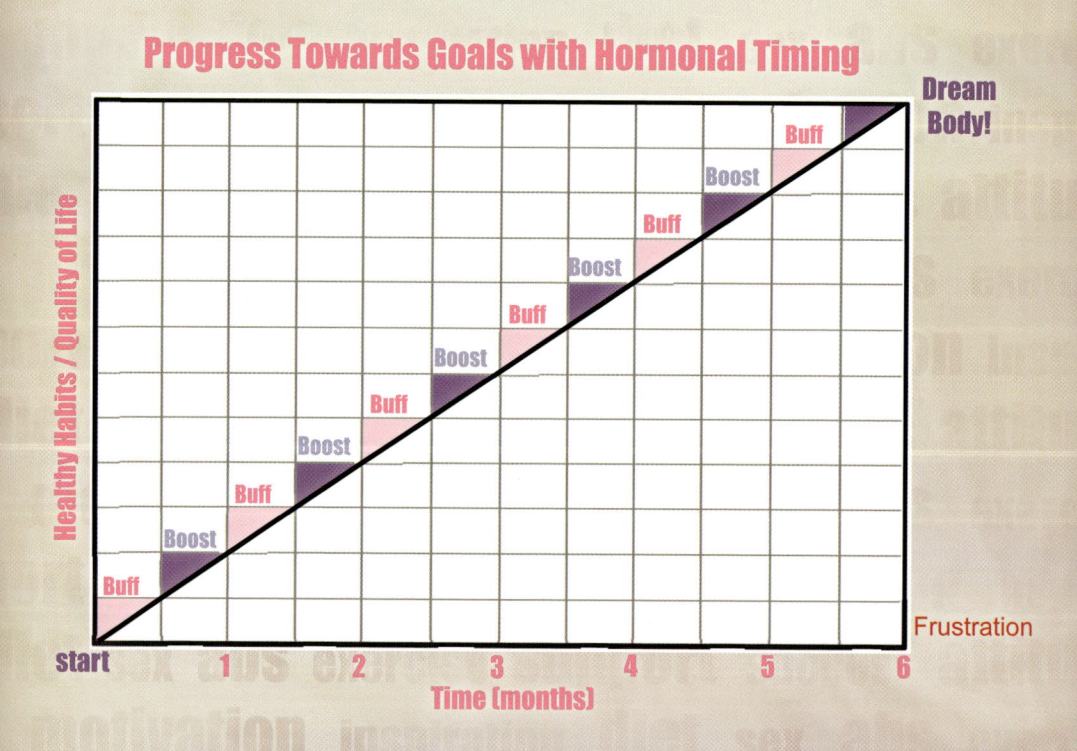

Progress Towards Goals with Hormonal Timing

Y-axis: Healthy Habits / Quality of Life
X-axis: Time (months) — start, 1, 2, 3, 4, 5, 6

Staircase progression: Buff, Boost, Buff, Boost, Buff, Boost, Buff, Boost, Buff, Boost, Buff → Dream Body!

Frustration

Harness the Power of your Hormones

"You can't describe Hormonal Timing, you must experience it!"

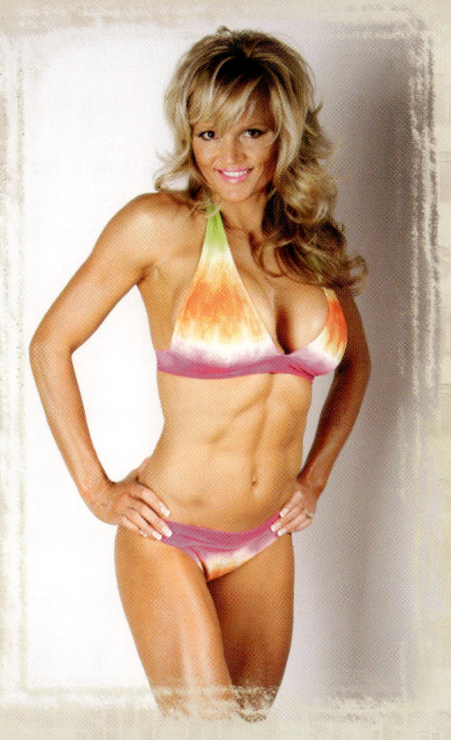

The graph below illustrates what happens to most women who follow a typical mainstream diet/fitness plan.

Progress Towards Goals with a Mainstream Program

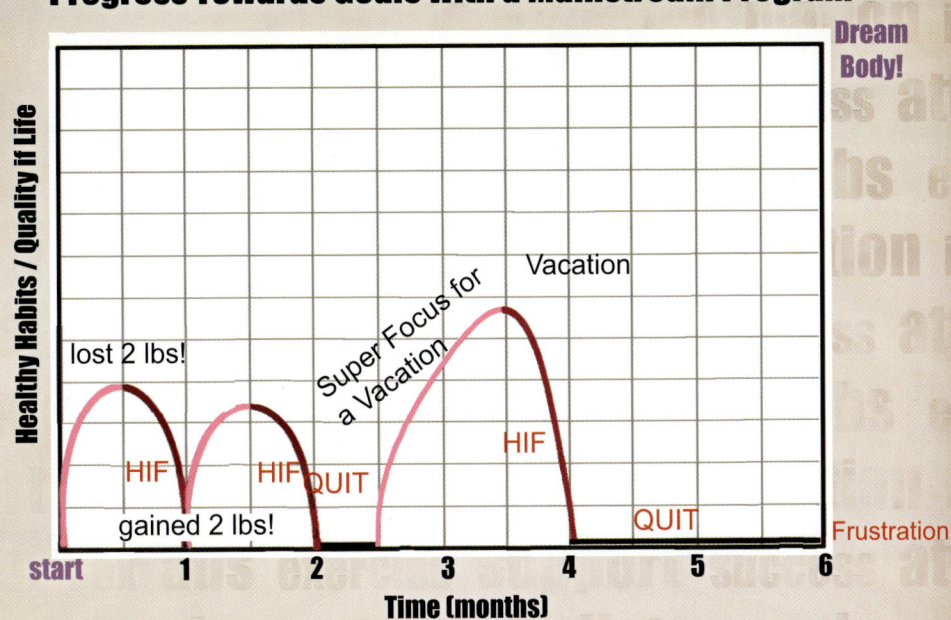

Healthy Habits / Quality if Life

lost 2 lbs!
HIF
HIF QUIT
gained 2 lbs!
Super Focus for a Vacation
Vacation
HIF
QUIT
Dream Body!
Frustration

start — 1 — 2 — 3 — 4 — 5 — 6
Time (months)

Harness the Power of your Hormones

47

Leslie's Testimony

Leslie Unterburger's fitness goals and challenges are a bit different than many of my clients. She wanted to have more curves and add some muscle to her "skinny fat" body. As a mother of 2 daughters, one of them being diabetic, Leslie knows the importance of being a good example to her kids. Leslie worked out for years without getting the results she desired but now on Hormonal Timing, Leslie is finally seeing the progress she craved. Utilizing the power of her hormones in the Boosting phase enabled her to finally regain her youthful shape. She is very excited to have her best body ever!

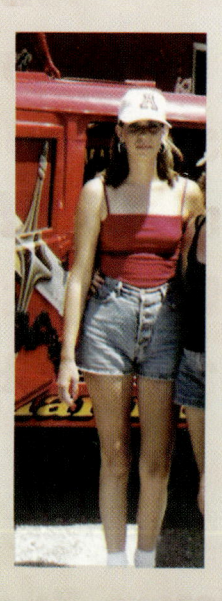

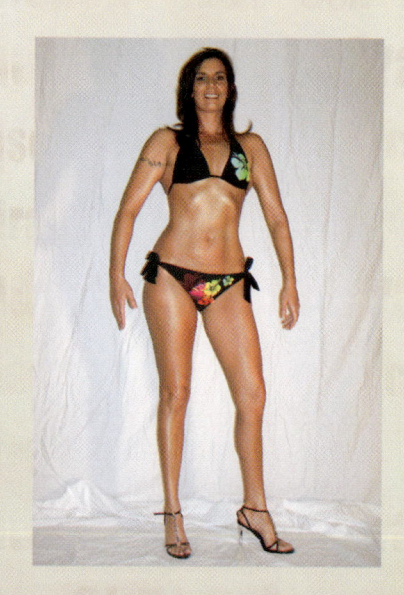

In her words....

I have always known that I get PMS symptoms every month. Cramps, bloating, irritability, sleepiness, you name it…It was responsible for sabotaging my fitness efforts.

Hormonal Timing, along with the supplements that Michelle recommends, have dramatically improved how I feel and how I perform. I think my "light bulb moment" was when I started counting my food portions. To my surprise, I was way low on portions and calories.

I think the key point about Hormonal Timing is it teaches us to recognize the pattern of changes that our bodies go through during our cycles and to work with that pattern to maximize our results from our fitness routines/diet. It is so much easier to work/achieve our goals when we "give ourselves a break" when our bodies need it. We don't need to deprive ourselves for the rest of our lives to look great! Hormonal Timing is something that is possible to do over a lifetime. I've broken a plateau that had been lingering too long! My results have been great!

Harness the Power of your Hormones

OK, we're off to a great start. You now understand:

1. "WHY" your hormones are the key to "Revolutionizing your BODY.
2. "HOW" to recognize when you are under attack from Hormone-Induced Failure (HIF).
3. "HOW" to calculate your cycle days and chart your hormones.
4. "WHAT" is happening inside your body relative to your hormones.
5. "HOW" to incorporate Buffing and Boosting into your life.

We have also covered the first 2 of the 10 Foundations
Foundation #1: Realize That You Are in a Battle!
Recognize when you are under attack and vulnerable for Hormone Induced Failure (HIF).

Foundation #2: Hormonal Timing - Use Hormonal Timing to capitalize on the good effects and negate the bad effects of your hormones

In section 5, titled "Nuts and Bolts for Action" (pg.79), I will give you a "turn key" fitness program that will get you on your way to your dream! But first we need to address your attitude, your belief, your reason, your motivation, your will….the next 5 Foundations center around your mentality. The most important factors for your success lie in your mind. No matter what "tools" (fitness plan, equipment, physical potential, money, etc) you have at your disposal, if your mind is unwilling to cooperate you won't be successful. With Hormonal Timing, you will experience a tremendous breakthrough simply from harnessing the power of your hormones, but I want to take you to the next level. It's now time to harness the power of your mind!

"I wanted 3 things: a sexy body, unlimited energy, and great kids! Hormonal Timing has allowed me to have it all!"

Harness the Power of your Hormones

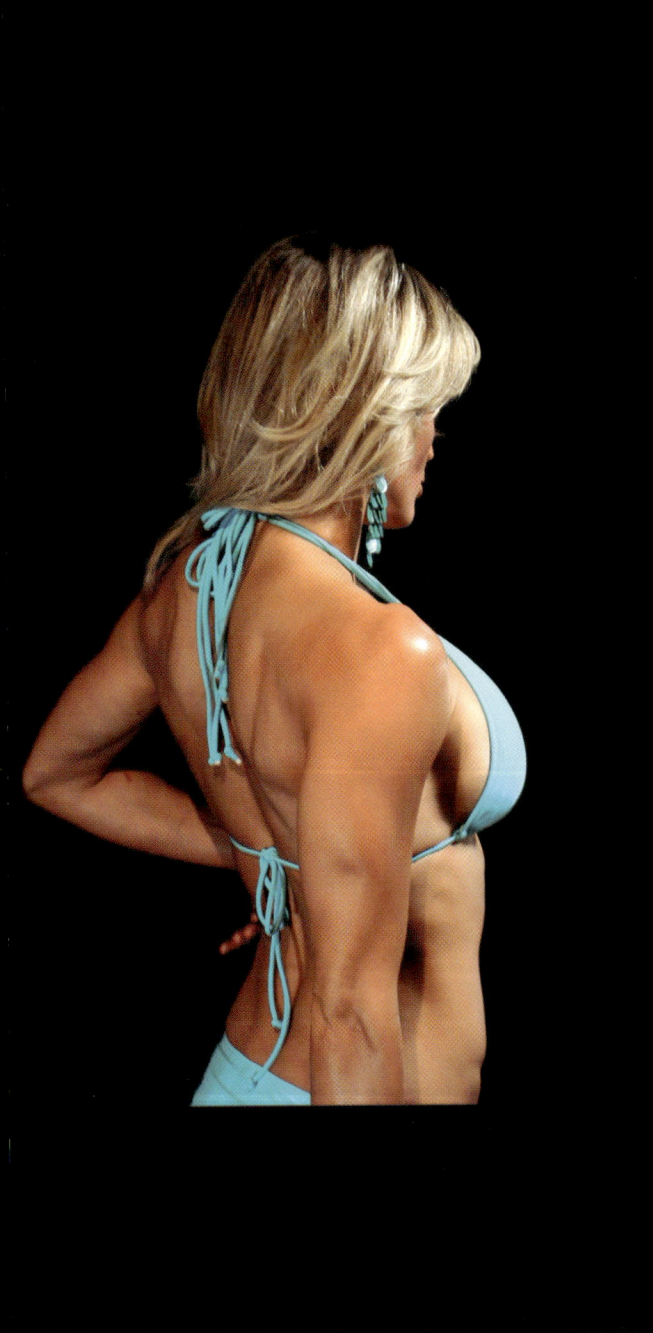

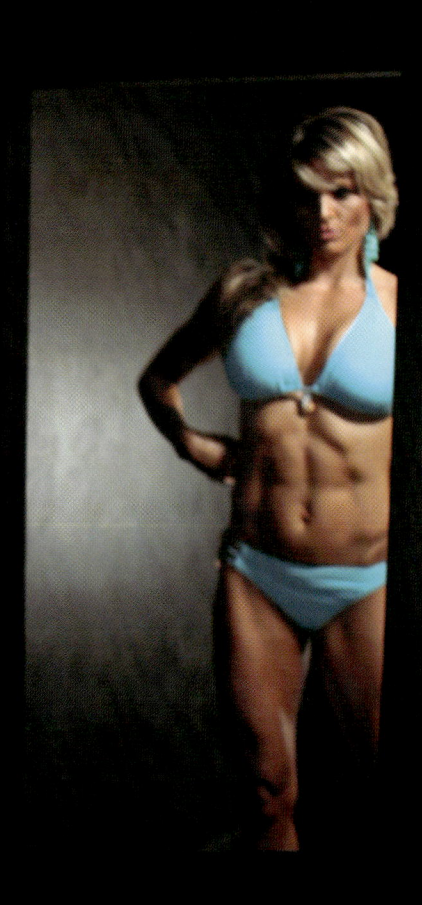

Train your Brain!

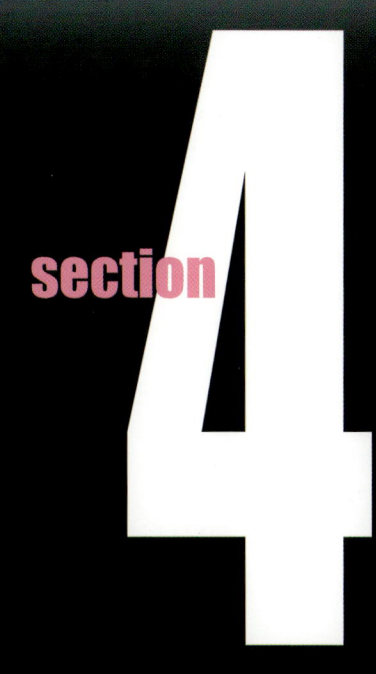

section 4

BELIEVE!

At least 90 percent of success is mental! I am constantly blown away by how true this is. I have witnessed it literally hundreds of times in the lives of my clients. I can always predict who will succeed and who will fail simply based on their willingness to work on developing the proper mentality. Training your brain is exactly like training any other body part. For example, let's say your legs are weak and you want to make them strong. If I was responsible for training you, I would begin by teaching you how to do lunges. At first, you will really struggle. Your leg muscles don't know what to do and you feel awkward and weak! After you recover for a few days, I will have you do them again. This time however, you feel a little stronger. Your legs have a little "muscle memory," so you're not as awkward and you don't struggle nearly as much as the first time. It doesn't take long before you start to almost enjoy doing them because you feel confident and strong. Every muscle will follow this very predictable pattern, and so will your mind! All you need to do is practice a few simple exercises and before long your mind will cooperate and be very strong!

Foundation #3: You Must Believe

I think the saying is "whether you believe you can or believe you can't you will be correct". I know this can be tough. After my twins were born, I remember looking in the mirror and being horrified by the sight of my stretched-out, saggy belly. Negative thoughts filled my head: "You're doomed! Stop wasting your time. Your abs are gone forever!" These thoughts created DOUBT in my mind. I was very discouraged and almost threw in the towel. However, I did have positive thoughts flash through my head as well. (Although not nearly as often or as loudly) Thoughts like: "You can do it! Keep working! Have a little faith!" Thankfully, I chose to listen to the positive thoughts. I took consistent action toward my goal of creating "better than ever" abs. I believed 100 percent that I would have awesome abs one day, and guess what? It happened!

There is a great verse in Mark chapter 9 of the BIBLE:
"Everything is possible for him who believes."
I live my life by this verse!

I wonder how many women fail simply because they choose to believe THOUGHTS OF DOUBT. My goal is to show you how to turn it all around with a very simple but extremely effective exercise. First, you must understand that DOUBT and BELIEF cannot co-exist. If you erase doubt you are left with belief and vice versa.

You must BELIEVE!
- Believe that your body is capable of the changes that you desire.
- Believe in the Hormonal Timing Lifestyle with all of your heart.
- Believe in yourself.
- Believe that you will accomplish your dreams.
- Keep saying, I BELIEVE_____....(you fill in the rest!)

Julie's Testimony
Julie's STORY is just AWESOME~ the words she wrote about believing say it all!! Julie has developed one of TEAM BuffMother's greatest leaders. She is constantly sharing her passion for fitness by working out with others, sharing tips with beginners and even giving speeches about her success! Over the last year I have witnessed her receiving great rewards from the energy she's given others. I am so proud to have such a generous person in my life!

Train your Brain

Julie a few years ago   Julie now

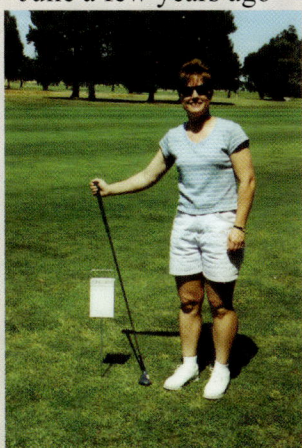

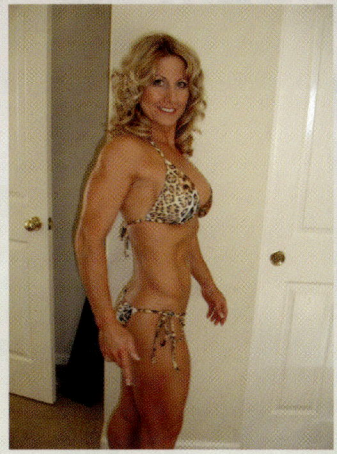

Here is what Julie wrote about her experience with her own belief:

In her words....

My name is Julie Laughrey and I'm a 47-year-young mother of 3 adult children. I had my first child at the age of 20 and my other two by the age of 26. I gave all I could to my children and their upbringing. I believed that I needed to put them first and I always put myself and my husband second. Then at the age of 39 something happened to me that changed the direction of my life as I knew it. I was diagnosed with fibromyalgia. My health became my number one goal. It was a lonely life, though, as none of my friends had this priority and they just didn't understand the new evolving me.

While surfing the web I found www.BuffMother.com, and life changed for me. As I was reading Michelle's introduction on "Believing" I realized that I was that mother that she was describing. I believed that if I tried to give myself that extra time in the day for ME to reach my desires that I would have been selfish. I had the belief that as you got older that you were just destined to look a certain way and age. This was a real light bulb moment. I realized that I wasted a lot of time and there was no more time to waste. I could achieve a new and improved me!

Since joining TEAM BuffMother, I finally got it. You can make changes and reach the goals that you set for yourself as long as you BELIEVE you can. I not only feel like this with my body now, but also with life in general. You can do anything you want and be anything you want. You just need to believe and you can achieve this and be a good mother, daughter, friend to others in the process. I now BELIEVE that I can do anything I set my mind to. I've learned to set fitness goals. I'd never really done that before. I've learned to set challenges for myself. I've been working out for many years, but with no real goals and no real diet. I now know how to fuel my workouts, how to CHALLENGE myself and receive the results that I'm looking for. As BuffMother! always says....Challenge=Change...I really BELIEVE that!!

Train your Brain

Success Tool #3- "Doubt Crushers"

The fastest way to build strong belief is to do a simple exercise called "DOUBT CRUSHERS." You don't even need to get off the couch for this exercise!

Here's how to do "Doubt Crushers":

- The instant any doubt enters your mind, CRUSH IT IMMEDIATELY with a predetermined positive thought. Think of it this way: Every doubt that enters your mind is a lie which must be "crushed" by the truth!
- For example, the simple act of looking at my reflection in the mirror made me DOUBT in my head that my body could ever look good again. Each time this DOUBT came to mind I would instantly say to myself, "I can do all things through Christ who strengthens me!!!" This phrase became my "truth hammer" and I bet I've used it at least 200,000 times over the last few years. I will continue to use it to eradicate doubt so that BELIEF can flourish in my life forever. I'll use it until the day I die!
- You can use any word phrase as long as it's positive, you believe it, and it's simple to remember. It can be as simple as saying "I believe," "just do it," "BuffMother UP!" "NO Excuses," etc... Just find one that really means something to you and use it relentlessly every time doubt enters your mind! See more examples on the next page.
- Crushing doubt is a <u>skill</u> which must be developed through consistent practice and dedication. You must practice using your "truth hammer"! At first you may need to write it all over your house, gym, mirrors, computer, etc....
- With practice, your "truth hammer" will automatically crush every doubt that dares to enter your mind. The key is to always have your favorite "truth hammer" on the tip of your tongue so you don't have any time to dwell on any doubt.

"Doubt Crushers"

truth hammer

DOUBT = BELIEF

You'll never get your body back...
You have to live with your new "MOMMY" body...
You'll never see your abs...

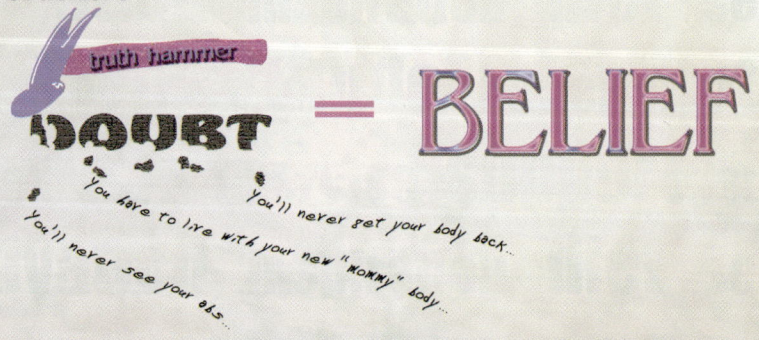

Train your Brain

Muscle burns fat

I need to fuel myself to perform

Muscle gives youthful shape to my body

I can...

Lifting weights reverses aging

Working out makes me feel GREAT!

I am driven...

Water Flushes the fat out

Keep a legacy perspective

It is the LITTLE things…

I am successful!

I can do all things...

I am creating a GREAT legacy~

I believe...

I am confident!

I am in control!

I am focused!

My body is responding!

This is working!

"Doubt Crushers" are very simple, but they are by no means easy. You need to practice them 24 hours a day 7 days a week for 30 days to assure total transformation. Don't let yourself dwell on any doubt! This exercise will yield immediate results, and before long you won't even notice you're doing it. Eventually, you will crush doubt automatically and unconsciously. When you get to that level, your belief will be unstoppable! **It is very important to select your positive affirmation or "truth hammer" right now**. Find one that really inspires you and say it over and over in your mind so it pops into your mind the second any doubt tries to show its ugly face! Do it now!!

Please write your favorite "truth hammers" here:

_____
_____
_____
_____
_____

You are now set to start crushing doubt, and be on the road to belief! Once you BELIEVE, the next aspect of your brain we must train is your ATTITUDE!

Foundation #4: PMA - All the Way, BABY!

"Always bear in mind that your own resolution to succeed is more important than any other one thing."- Abraham Lincoln

This is a very powerful quote from one of the most successful men in American history. His life was filled with one failure after another until he finally triumphed and become President of the United States.

Entire books have been written on the FACT that having a positive mental attitude (PMA) is absolutely crucial if you want to succeed at anything. I have to admit that I'm a recovering "bad attitudaholic." I've had numerous setbacks in my life that have totally derailed me from reaching my goals. Many times these were merely "speed bumps," but when you mix a speed bump with a bad attitude, you create a gigantic mountain. I've come to the realization that no matter how hard I try, I can't always control what happens to me. In life there will always be adversity. However, I do have total control over how I react to it. That's the key! YOU ALWAYS HAVE CONTROL OVER YOUR ATTITUDE! You can do it. You can have a PMA!!

Have you ever tried to just "have a positive attitude?" Some people make is sound so easy. I've heard people say "Have a positive attitude about it!" That works for about 9 seconds and then BAM, it turns right back into negative! Truthfully, I think it's impossible to simply change your negative attitude into a positive attitude permanently. It's like trying to change a duck into a chicken. Dress it up anyway you want but at the end of the day, a duck is a duck!

However, there is a way to "turn your frown upside down" permanently. The long-term solution is to change your FOCUS! The reason most people have attitude problems is because they are constantly focused on the problem. They think about the problem, worry about the problem, talk about the problem, write about the problem, complain about the problem, etc. Have you ever caught yourself doing this; You give all of your strength and energy to your problem until you are physically and mentally exhausted? I've done it many times and I know it's a recipe for failure. The more energy you give to a problem the bigger it will become.

Here's a fact:
"Problem focused" women always end up discouraged, depressed, helpless and worst of all HOPELESS! When all hope has been lost they are left with complete and utter misery.

How would you like to wake up every day with a PMA?
Here's how...

    A great strategy for creating an eternal PMA is to focus all of your energy on <u>SOLUTIONS instead of your problems!</u> It's really very simple, but at first it won't be easy. From now on, you will be the "fixer" in your own life. Every problem has a solution and it's your job to find it! You might need to test 100 different possible solutions before finally finding one that works. The point is that you are pouring all of your energy into brainstorming for solutions and then testing them by taking immediate action. This will create a tidal wave of hope in your life. It's easy to maintain a PMA if you are always overflowing with hope.

    Being "Solution Focused" will create hope and lead to a life filled with PMA.

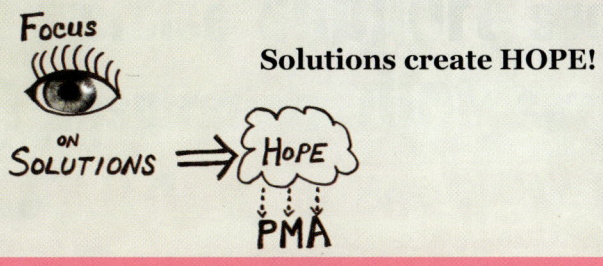

Solutions create HOPE!

Success Tool #4- Focus on Solutions!

    Take out a sheet of paper. At the top, write down an obstacle/problem you are currently facing. Next, brainstorm and write down every possible solution. Now tear the problem off the top of the paper, crumple it up and get rid of it. I suggest burning it, but it's not a must. The point is you must totally forget about the problem. Mentally focus all of your energy on every possible solution. Then, begin acting on the solutions. You will find that even though your problem might still exist, it doesn't have power over you. Instead, all of your energy is pouring into solutions. The feeling you now have is called HOPE, and it's the only thing that can fuel long term PMA.

Focusing on <u>solutions</u> creates <u>hope</u> which fuels a <u>PMA</u>.

1. Write the problem or obstacle at the top of a sheet of paper.
2. List the all the possible solutions.
3. Eliminate problem (tear off, burn it and forget it). Give no time, energy or focus to it at all!!
4. Give 100 percent FOCUS towards the solutions- keep the solutions in front of you constantly, read them, think about them and HOPE will explode!
5. PMA will now grow.

Train your Brain

How I used **"Focus on Solutions™!"** to create my ABS:

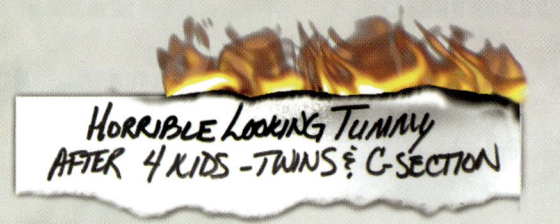

> HORRIBLE LOOKING TUMMY
> AFTER 4 KIDS - TWINS & C-SECTION

Trash or Burn the Problem!

> EVERY POSSIBLE SOLUTION:
> SUCK IT IN
> DO "ABS" DAILY - THROUGH PAIN
> DO THE HARDEST AB EXERCISES - SITUPS
>   ROMAN CHAIR
> DO VACUUMS
> DO CATS
> DO OTHER LIFTING WORKOUTS
> DO CARDIO - INTERVALS - SPRINTS
> DIET!! EAT PROTEIN & GREENS
> NO DAIRY, CARBONATION, SWEETNERS
> HYDRATE - WATER & LOTION!!
> SUPPLEMENTS!

Focus on SOLUTIONS™!

I focused on the solutions (still do) and went from being disgusted by my tummy to having hope about the potential of my tummy and now through my success have been able to give HOPE to other mothers! My being focused on solutions allowed me to have PMA which in turn has created an enormous amount of energy in the world. Mothers are energized to take action… which energized me to keep working hard until the day I die. Let me now share my secret of how you can experience the phenomenon I call Exponential Energy™!

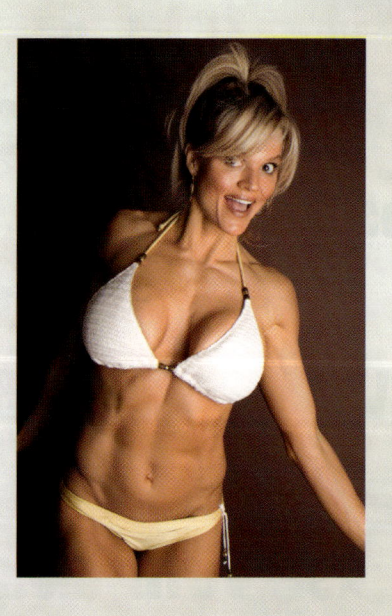

Train your Brain

How to Create Exponential Energy™

Now it's time to introduce you to one of my "secret weapons." I believe it's the key to turning your dreams, goals, desires, etc., into reality! How do I know? Because I tested it myself, and it worked! In fact, it continues to work more and more every day in my life and it will for you too! **Have you ever considered how much energy is contained in one little seed?**

Consider the energy contained in a single acorn:
- If you plant an acorn it can grow into a huge oak tree.
- That oak tree can produce thousands more acorns.
- Those acorns can grow into a huge forest.
- That forest can be converted into millions of tons of lumber.
- That lumber can be used to build an entire kingdom!
- I could go on and on but the fact is, there are no limits to what can be produced from a single acorn!!!

There are no limits to what can grow from a single seed! This is a natural law of the universe. It applies to everything and is mind-boggling when you think about it.

Every thought, deed, action, comment, idea, etc., is a seed filled with potential energy that can grow and multiply.

What does this have to do with Health & Fitness? Everything!

I vividly remember an incident that took place at the gym one day that made me discover the power of planting a single positive seed! I had recently resumed my workouts after having my twins and the going was rough. My motivation level was low and I was very tired! I was 100 percent focused on myself. I didn't feel like socializing with anyone in any way. I just wanted to enjoy a little time to myself while the gym childcare staff watched my 4 little ones. I remember looking up and noticing someone who looked familiar. She appeared to be leaner than the last time I saw her and looked much better. I didn't know her and I'd never spoken to her before, but I suddenly felt compelled to tell her how great she looked. I took the focus off of myself, walked across the gym and said, "I can tell you've been working hard because you look great!" She was floored! As it turns out, she had been going through some struggles and really needed to hear exactly what I had to say that day. Her reaction caught me completely off guard and really blew me away! I felt a rush of energy that was absolutely pure. It was a kind of energy that you can't get from caffeine. It can't be put in a bottle or pill. This form of energy can only be experienced by practicing the 5th foundational principle.

Foundation #5: Energize Others

You have been blessed with very unique talents, gifts, abilities, opportunities, ideas, thoughts, etc. These can all be described as seeds of energy and nobody on earth, past, present, or future will have access to the same combination of these seeds as you!

Every one of these **"energy seeds"** can be planted and exponentially multiply exactly like the acorn example. However, you must learn to take the focus off yourself and use these seeds to energize others without expecting anything in return!

"You can have anything in the world you want if you'll just help enough other people get what they want." -Zig Ziglar

Consider the energy contained in a single "energy seed":
- If you plant an "energy seed" it can inspire another to action
- That action creates more "energy seeds" and may produce hundreds more inspired actions
- The energy continues to grow at an exponential rate, building upon each person's inspired actions along the way planting more "energy seeds." EXPONENTIAL ENERGY™ is created!
- The fact is there are no limits to what can be produced by planting an "energy seed". Plant your "energy seeds" NOW!!! You will be rewarded with EXPONENTIAL ENERGY!

Another way to put it is to GIVE away what you have. Have you ever heard the expression, "It is more blessed to give than receive"? This verse comes from the book of Acts in the Bible. Virtually every religion and or philosophical viewpoint teaches about the importance of giving. Personally, I can't say that I was inspired or enthused in any way when I first read about giving to others. I didn't feel I had anything to give and what I did have I needed for myself! You might feel the same way. However, I now believe that nothing has more power to unleash incredible rewards into your life than the act of giving to benefit other people!

Identify your Gifts, Passion, and Talents

Now let's take it one step further.....In order to give, you must know what you have to give. In the exact same way that everyone has needs, every person also has been blessed with certain gifts, talents and abilities. **These gifts are your "energy seeds"!!!**

Train your Brain

Write down every gift, talent, skill, ability, or thing you like doing or are good at.
For example:
I am good at writing.
I have always been a great encourager.
I love organizing things.
I am generous.
I enjoy manual labor.
I have excellent computer skills.

Can you imagine what will happen in your life if you decide to "plant" your gifts into the lives of others? In time you will experience what can only be described as a natural phenomenon. The energy from every seed you planted will multiply exponentially and flow back to you! It's so simple, but you need to be willing to take the first step. Don't sit around thinking, talking and worrying about the things you don't have. Instead, use what you do have to help other people (plant your "energy seeds") In time, you will always be rewarded exponentially!!

Energize Others
For the next 30 days I want you to energize others by planting (giving) energy. You will experience 2 benefits;
1. You will feel instant gratification when you sincerely help someone in need. Giving **always** feels far better than you originally predicted.
2. Sooner or later, a tidal wave of energy will flow into your life. Every need you have will miraculously be met. Don't try to figure out how it works. Just go DO IT NOW and find out for yourself!!

**There is one little catch. You must give without expecting anything in return! If you only "give" to "get," this law won't have any power in your life and you will be completely wasting your time!

Now that you know what you have to give (your personal "energy seeds")... **WHO** do you give them to? We all know that walking up to a stranger at the gym and giving a compliment is not an easy thing to do. Sometimes finding someone who openly wants and is willingly to accept a genuine act of kindness is the hardest part of planting "energy seeds." Well, I have the simplest solution; We've created the perfect place where a bunch of really great women get together to plant positive "energy seeds" in each other's lives. We've named this place the Rally Room!

Success Tool #5- The Rally Room...A "Field of Dreams"!!!

The Rally Room is a place you can go where the sole purpose is to use your gifts to help other women. The power that is released in that place is indescribable! This little "secret society" or team is located online in a very secure section of www.BuffMother.com. Everyone brings their own brand of positive energy to the team and they receive an explosion of positive energy in return. You can never out give this team!

Many women in the Rally Room (RR) had tried every imaginable way to stay motivated. The mainstream fitness gurus have advised numerous methods to keep women motivated: reading magazines, visualizing, hiring a trainer, goal setting, etc., but none of them are effective long term. However, the ladies in the Rally Room have discovered the **secret**. The key to unlocking this motivational mystery, the secret to staying motivated is to <u>forget about yourself long enough to encourage someone else!</u> That's right; All you need to do is plant "energy seeds" among the women in the RR in a sincere and genuine way. You will be amazed at what will happen when you make a habit out of doing this. Your motivation to stick to your own goals skyrockets! Encouraging someone else doesn't have to be saying "you can do it." It can be done in so many other ways. You can find a million ways to use your gifts in the RR to help other women. The sky is the limit and everyone in there will welcome you with open arms. It's awesome!!

How to use the Rally Room as your Success tool to create EXPONENTIAL ENERGY!

A Basic Step-by-Step:
1. Sign up to the Rally Room through www.BuffMother.com
2. Create your profile, share as much information as you can about yourself in your profile...it will help you "connect" with other women just like you.
3. Read through some other members' profiles and blogs. You will find many women that will quickly become close friends.
4. Start planting "energy seeds"...the easiest most gratifying way to do this is to comment on another member's blog.
   - Write what you are thinking with the most positive spin you can create in words.
   - Simply typing "hi" makes that teammate feel special. It lets them know they are important.
   - If you see someone struggling in an area you've overcome, take them under your wing and share with them what you've learned.

Train your Brain

5. If encouraging someone sounds daunting or hard…please glance through the following list of actions that are basically "energy seeds." Pick 1 or 2 of them that you are excited about and start "planting" them in the Rally Room.

Accept	Design	Guide	Promote
Accommodate	Detail	Happy	Prompt
Advise	Develop	Harmonize	Recommend
Advocate	Discipline	Help	Rescue
Affirm	Discover	Identify	Research
Analyze	Donate	Impact	Respond
Assemble	Dramatize	Implement	Schedule
Assist	Edify	Improve	Search
Assure	Empathize	Improvise	See opportunity
Avoid hurting	Encourage	Influence	Selfless
Befriend	Endow	Inspire	Shoulder
Build up	Enforce	Interpret	Show kindness
Carry through	Enjoys	Lead	Show mercy
Caution	Enlighten	Lecture	Solve
Challenge	Entertainer	Lover	Stimulate
Checks facts	Envision	Maintain	Strengthen
Cheer up	Establish	Minister	Studies
Cherish	Evangelize	Modify	Supervise
Coach	Evoke	Moralize	Support
Comfort	Examine	Motivate	Sustain
Command	Experiment	Nurture	Sympathize
Communicate	Explore	Observe	Talk
Convict	Expose	Organize	Teach
Coordinate	Feel	Overcome	Testify
Correct	Follow up	Perform	Train
Counsel	Forewarn	Persevere	Trust
Create	Forgive	Persist	Unify
Cultivate	Formulate	Persuade	Urge
Decide	Give	Pioneer	Work hard
Delegate	Goal oriented	Prescribe	Write
Demonstrate	Govern	Proclaim	

6. Keep it going~ remember that you will have down times, busy times and times when your hormones may cause you to become less confident, energetic or positive. When you feel this (often during Boosting), make an extra effort to continue on in planting seeds of energy. You will reap a bountiful garden of exponential energy soon!

Train your Brain

Rally Room Expectations:

In the Rally Room we have 3 simple rules: no men allowed, PG-rated content only and keep a POSITIVE tone. The third rule exists because there is a flip side to this Universal Law that I need to warn you about: If you choose to plant "negative" seeds, you will experience negative results! This was a huge revelation to me; **If I release negative energy it will circle back on me!** This means that if I say something bad about someone behind their back, I will be repaid with something negative in the future! Many women completely transform their lives simply by making the decision to say something nice or say nothing at all. My advice when tempted to criticize, condemn or complain, BITE YOUR TONGUE!! You will never regret NOT saying something bad.

Cara's Testimony

Cara has a way of putting a big grin on my face. This lovely woman admits she felt alone and had very low self esteem prior to being a member of TEAM BuffMother. From her involvement in the RR, I have personally witnessed the changes in her. She has become a positive, courageous and confident woman. Her attitude has spilled over into other areas of her life. She stepped out and started her own business and now has big plans for her future. Reading her testimony about the Rally Room was a GREAT experience!! I loved her key points: The fact that the Rally Room is like a family, that there is almost a magical effect in encouraging others and in knowing there is a TEAM behind you giving you strength to take on the challenges of life!

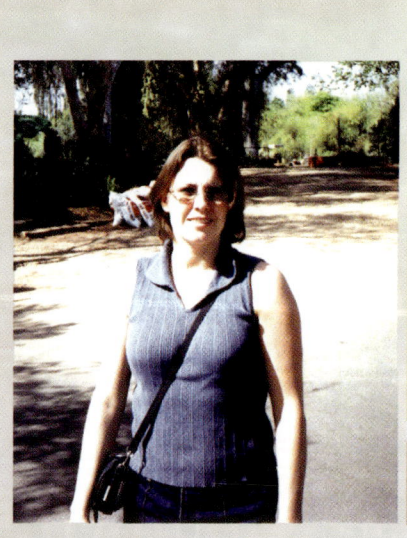

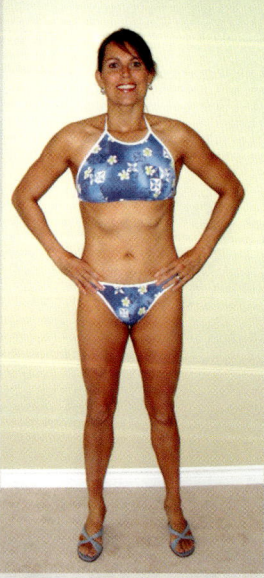

Cara's Awesome essay on Why She LOVES the Team BuffMother! Rally Room...

In her words....

Prior to joining the Rally Room, I was somewhat isolated due to having a new baby. In fact, I was often lonely and felt like no one outside of my family really cared about me. My good friends had moved away and the acquaintances that were nearby didn't have a passion for health and fitness. I had no one other than my immediate family to share my aspirations with. I felt as though no one understood why I would want to spend my time working out to create an ultimate physique rather than "enjoying life". I began searching for something that would fuel the flame for my love of health and fitness and support my efforts. Well, I found it in the hidden gem of the Rally Room and everything has changed since then.

To give you a clearer picture of what it is like in the Rally Room, I would like to pose to you the following question. Have you ever been in a room full of people and felt as though you were among family? Well, that is how I feel when I am in the Rally Room. I can let my inhibitions down, speak my mind and find comfort knowing that the other women understand my trials and triumphs whether it is related to my workouts or personal issues. The Rally Room is my sanctuary. I feel a sense of pride knowing that I am part of something "BIG." I am proud to be a part of a group of women that make a difference in each others' lives by providing advice, encouragement and most importantly friendship. Over the months, I have come to know many of the women on a personal level through reading and responding to individual blogs. This has been very fulfilling for me. I feel as though my opinions are valued and that I have a purpose in the Rally Room. On the flip side, the countless women who have lifted me up and made me feel special by responding to my blogs are unbelievable. Their responses really encourage me to keep going. I don't want to let myself down and more importantly I don't want to let the girls down. I have a new mindset and dedication to my workouts since joining the Rally Room.

I do owe some of my success to Michelle's program and her expertise; however, I must give credit to the other women who have given me encouragement and some great tips along the way. It is amazing how the support of others helps you reach your goals. I can't even imagine what life would be like without my daily dose of the BuffMother Rally Room. As I like to say, "One week without the Rally Room makes one weak." I am confident that others will love this place as much as I do. - Cara of Canada, mother of 2

"The definition of regret is when the person you are meets the person you could be!"

Train your Brain

"The Key to Your Motivation…"

3 common factors that can affect your motivation level:

1) **Your Hormones-** As previously discussed, your hormone fluctuations can have a dramatic affect on whether or not you have inner drive to get after it! Hormonal Timing will solve this issue once and for all!

2) **Lack of Support-** You might feel like you're "all alone" in your quest to get in shape and practice healthy habits. The Rally Room is a great tool if this is how you feel. It is full of like-minded women from around the world. You may not have personal friends who are willing to support you and you may live in an area where there doesn't seem to be a "healthy" person in sight! However, if you tap into the Rally Room, you will connect with a family that will do whatever it takes to help you succeed!!

3) **Your Why-** You may be suffering from a "weak why." In my experience, this may be the most common reason that so many women feel flat-out unmotivated! Answer this question; Why did you buy your last diet pill, weight loss system, exercise device, etc? Most women say, "to lose weight". In fact, most women are obsessed with losing weight and this often leads to failure. If your mission revolves solely around losing weight, you will struggle when times get tough!

Evaluate YOUR "WHY" …Why Am I Doing This?!?!?!

You will subconsciously ask yourself this question thousands of times throughout your fitness journey. Every time you are faced with a "good vs. evil" choice, your subconscious wants to know "is it worth it"? Believe it or not, success or failure could depend on the strength of your "WHY." This is the scenario; you had planned to get some exercise after work. However, when you get home, you feel sore, tired and grumpy. Here comes the question: "WHY am I doing this again?" Followed by: "Is it really worth it?" Your CHOICE will depend on the strength of your "WHY".

Other common scenarios:
- When your diet calls for a green veggie but you want to eat cookies….WHY…?
- When you need to get up and exercise but the couch suddenly feels so comfy…WHY…?
- When you want to complain about something but you know you should choose a PMA….WHY…?

Do you have a "WEAK WHY"? Let's test it!

Most women will answer the "WHY" question with one of the following;
- I need to lose weight!
- I want to wear the same size as I did in college!
- I want to look more attractive!

Train your Brain

These are all great <u>REASONS</u> to practice healthy habits but they are what I call "WEAK WHYS." They might work for a short time but they simply aren't strong enough to help you make good choices on a permanent basis.

A STRONG WHY vs A WEAK WHY

The following exercise will demonstrate the dramatic differences between the two...Please put some effort into this so you can really "feel" the impact!

1) A WEAK WHY

I want you to imagine that you are standing on the roof of a very tall skyscraper. The wind is gusting so hard that you're scared you might be blown right off the building! As you look around, you notice a very long, narrow plank that leads to another skyscraper. Then you notice that the second skyscraper is engulfed in flames! Your mind is spinning because it's all happening so fast!

Suddenly a man appears and presents you with a once-in-a-lifetime opportunity. He tells you that if you are willing to risk your life and walk across the narrow plank to the burning building, you will instantly attain every **visible** and/or **measurable** physical change you have ever desired. This means instantly losing that "10, 30 or 80 pounds" or suddenly wearing a size 2 dress! It can be anything you want as long as it involves a physical transformation which is **visible** and or **measurable** in some way (scale, tape measure, dress size, etc). All you need to do is cross over to the roof of the burning building and you will have them! Remember, the wind is blowing at gale force and the plank is narrow. You need to make a decision fast before the building collapses! What choice do you make? I'm guessing that you are tempted by the offer but in the end you decline. Physical transformation is just not enough to make you risk your life. A "why" that is based solely on visible, measurable physical change is WEAK!

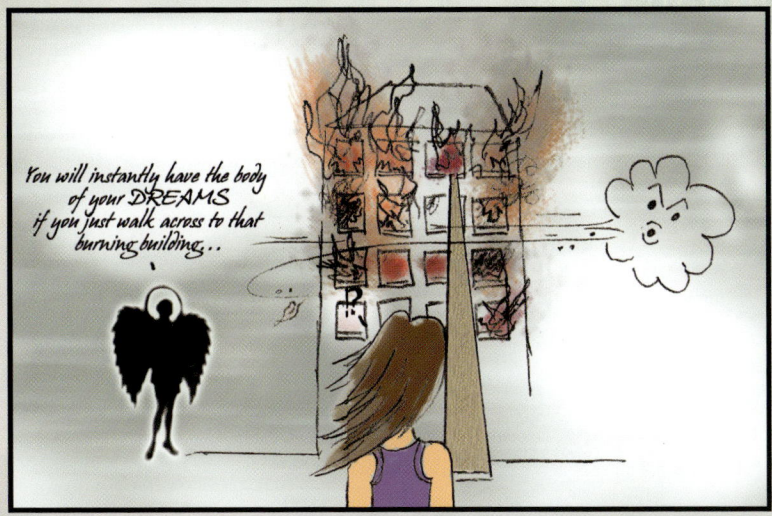

2) A STRONG WHY

Let's use the same scenario to illustrate the power of a "STRONG WHY."

You are back on top of the skyscraper and all of the same conditions are in effect. Gale force winds, narrow plank, burning skyscraper, etc. However, this time as you gaze over at the flaming building you notice something that sends you into an uncontrollable frantic panic. You see your children standing in the burning building. They are waving at you and screaming "MOMMY SAVE US!!"

What do you do? The answer is obvious; you throw caution to the wind and race across to save your babies! This is the definition of a "STRONG WHY"! The difference is staggering, isn't it?

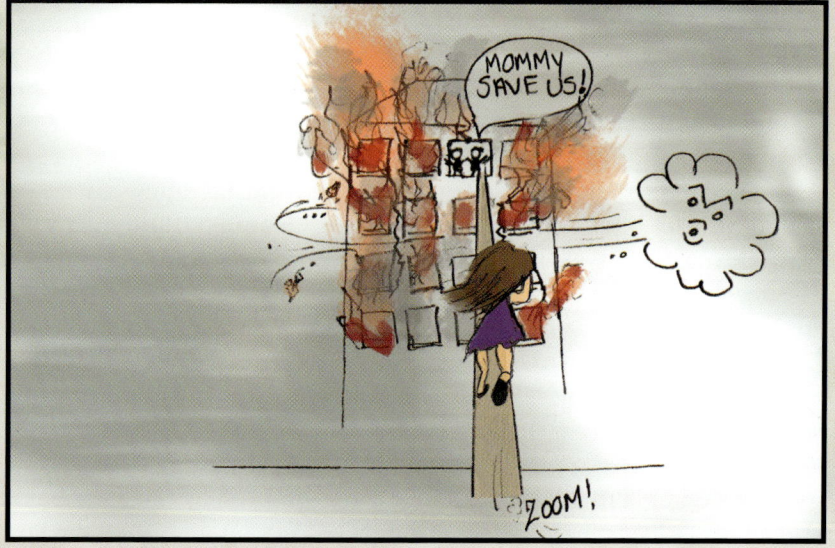

The Mainstream Diet industry is responsible for creating "WEAK WHYS"

Please understand; the vast majority of all Diet and Fitness companies are focused on one thing; MAKING MONEY! I'm sure many of them genuinely care about helping people but make no mistake, they are PROFIT driven. As a result, they spend millions of dollars to convince us that their products will deliver FASTER, EASIER, EFFORTLESS, etc, results. If one company says you can lose 20 lbs in 30 days the next company says you can lose 20 lbs in 25 days! They are all racing to develop products that claim "faster and easier" results!

Here's the problem: These diet companies always measure success in terms of immediate weight loss or "inches lost" or some other visible, measurable result!

This focus on fast, easy weight loss sets us up for failure because the truth is; dramatic results take work, discipline, sacrifice, discomfort, etc. You need a better reason than "losing weight" to justify paying the price of success. You won't experience the euphoric success that Hormonal Timing has to offer, until you develop a "STRONG WHY."

Train your Brain

Foundation #6: Live with a LEGACY Perspective!!

Living with a Legacy perspective creates a "STRONG WHY"!

1) Take the focus off of yourself. Forget about your weight, dress size, body fat percentage, etc. You will be rewarded with all of these physical changes but don't focus on them right now!

2) Focus on your LEGACY! The fact is, whether we like it or not, we are all creating a legacy right now! This legacy will affect our children, grandchildren, and on and on…

The choices we make today will impact future generations of our families. This can be either exciting or depressing depending on our daily habits.

Two kinds of Legacies

You will either leave a POSITIVE legacy or a NEGATIVE legacy! Every action leaves an IMPRINT. Simply ask yourself "will this leave a positive imprint or negative"??? Furthermore, you will leave an imprint on every person with whom you come into contact. Family, friends, co-workers, casual acquaintances and even people you meet one time and never see again. YOU WILL LEAVE AN IMPRINT ON EVERYONE!! Your legacy will be defined by the combined affect of these millions and millions of imprints. Simply reading this book leaves an imprint that will last forever!

I want you take a minute and think about how you were affected by previous generations. Generally speaking, if your mother had a great attitude, she probably passed it on to you. The same goes for her diet choices and exercise habits. However, the vast majority of us did <u>not</u> have mothers with great attitudes, who ate healthfully and exercised regularly. Most women can't even remember seeing their mothers exercise at all. The only memories most of have is when our mothers tried some horrible crash diet, felt miserable, complained about "the scale" and how impossible it was to lose weight! These attitudes, beliefs, actions and reactions are **imprinted** on us and they are difficult to erase. We are products of what we witnessed growing up. Furthermore, we continue to pass along these generational "curses" no matter how much we love our children and those around us.

"There are only 2 kinds of Legacies: negative and positive. There are varying degrees, but you must understand that it is impossible to leave behind a "NEUTRAL" legacy."

Train your Brain

I'm sure we can all agree that the thought of creating a negative legacy is horrifying. I doubt that any mother would consciously try to create this type of legacy. Unfortunately, it is <u>happening right now in millions of American families.</u>

Case in point: Childhood obesity is at epidemic levels despite the hundreds of millions that is being spent to stop it. The only possible solution is in the hands of the most powerful group of people in the world. The group I'm referring to is us! That's right, **MOTHERS!** We need to rise up and take action!

....Let's go back to the burning building situation with a slight modification. It's not just your child standing on that building yelling "MOMMY!" It's every future child that will be born into your family! Your choices will live on and will have a dramatic effect on them even if you never meet them!! I'm assuming that every woman reading this book wants to leave an Ultra-POSITIVE LEGACY. You want your family, friends, co-workers, and all future generations to say things like:

- "My mom is an incredible woman; she changed her attitude, transformed her body and became unstoppable!"
- "I want to be just like her! She is always so happy."
- "Every time I talk to her, I feel energized."
- "She has incredible self confidence."
- Your great-great grandma was an all star!

Here's the GREAT NEWS: You have total control over every aspect of your legacy! The past doesn't matter. It's never too late to change your legacy! NEVER!!! Starting today the slate has been wiped clean. You have the opportunity to make a fresh start beginning now. **You have the power to create a positive legacy for your family!**

The great benefit of living with a legacy perspective is if we are successful in attaining <u>this</u> incredible goal, we will automatically be blessed with every other desire we originally wanted:
- Weight loss
- Great body
- Boundless energy
- Incredible self confidence
- Extremely high self-esteem
- Awesome sex life
- Etc…

OK so how do we start building a positive legacy?
Let's start with a very powerful exercise that can change your life…

Train your Brain

Success Tool #6- The 24 Hour Legacy Test

Imagine that today is your last day on Earth. Your entire legacy will be based solely on the imprints you leave behind TODAY. If you are a mother, your children will model their behavior based on what they see you do or not do TODAY.

That's right, you have just 24 hours and your children will mimic every imprint you leave behind. They will also pass these imprints on to their children and so on…your legacy from this one day will live on forever in future generations!!!

For this ONE DAY:
What will your attitude be like? Circle one:
    Bad/Negative
    Same as usual
    Unstoppable
Will your children hear you complain?
Will you make excuses all day?
Will you show anger toward anyone?
What will you choose to eat?_____
Will they see you take even 5 minutes to exercise?
Will you hug your children/husband?
How many times will you say "I love you"?
What kind of language will you use?
Will you say things that encourage those around you?
Will your focus be on you or will it be on those you love?
Will you focus on positive things or negative things?
Will you sit on the couch and watch TV?
Will your kids see you drink water? Coke? Beer/wine?
Will they hear you laugh?
Will you take a few minutes to show them how to work hard on something?

Was this 24 hour period extremely different than your normal day? Did the "legacy perspective" have an influence on your thoughts and test answers? You must realize the incredible power you have to influence future generations simply based on the choices you make on a daily basis. Everything leaves an eternal imprint!

Think of the huge payoff here!!! You can have a positive impact on your great, great, great, grandchildren simply by making positive little choices each day. Every good decision you make from today until you die will benefit your family for generations to come. You have TOTAL CONTROL over the most important aspects of your Legacy. **Imagine how incredible your life would be if you lived every single day according to your answers on this 24 HOUR LEGACY TEST!!**

Train your Brain

In order for this point to really "hit home" here are a few cool stories used as illustrations. These stories are from real women regarding how their positive choices have impacted their children, how they were affected by their mothers' choices, and how they have made many sacrifices, from a health and fitness standpoint, which have paid off years later in their children's lives.

In her words....

Jenn with her girls:

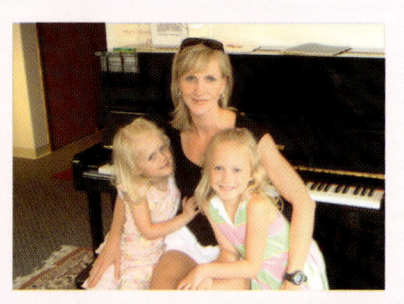

I grew up eating anything and everything I possibly wanted as a kid (mostly sugar, sugar and more sugar). My mother has always been very overweight and has had a lot of health problems because of her obesity. I decided at a very early age that I would never let myself be like that and that I would be a good example to my kids.

My resolve has kept me very active and fit all my life. I even continued to run and lift weights until the very end with both pregnancies. Fitness is a HUGE part of my life and a priority. My children realize that mommy works out every day, and that it is important to exercise and eat healthy to have the best life. Now I have two little runners who love to exercise with mommy. When I take my kids to the park my 5-year-old and I always do chin-ups and climb the poles together. My 5-year-old likes me to time her to see how long it takes to go across the monkey bars.

My little girls love to show me their "muscles" and are very aware of nutritional labels. My 5-year-old reads the labels and tells me how many grams of sugar, protein, etc. a product has. I am happy to say I broke the cycle of obesity with my girls. I am raising two health-conscious, fit kids.

In her words....

April with her son:

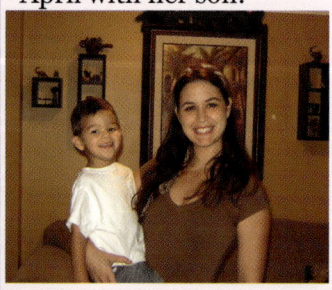

My son is 2 now and my husband and I have been working out since before he was born, so his whole life he was in the gym with us. Before he could walk, he'd watch us in his swing or car seat. And now that he's older, he walks on the treadmill with us and he lifts his own little 3lb dumbbell and goes "ungghh" just like his mom and dad do! So it just goes to show you, even when they're that young, you can still set an example to be healthy! Also when it comes to sweets, he prefers fruit over candy because he sees mom eating it all the time!

Train your Brain

Your WHY!- Summary:

- A "weak why" will eventually be defeated.
- If your "why" revolves solely around your weight, size, looks, or any other measured visible result, you will not experience long-term phenomenal success.
- A "STRONG WHY" is critical for achieving big time success!! And, it must revolve around the people you love.
- Understand that your choices will leave eternal imprints on your family.
- Realize that you control every critical factor in creating a positive Legacy. You are in a powerful position!
- Foundation #6-Living your life with a "Legacy Perspective" will result in success in other areas such as weight loss, more energy, etc...
- Success tool #6- the 24-hour Legacy Test, really puts things in proper perspective.

I know all this "legacy" stuff might sound daunting, overwhelming, impossible, etc. You might be thinking, "How do I even begin to change my legacy"?

It's really very simple. It's sort of like the question, "How do you eat an elephant?" That's right, ONE BITE AT A TIME!

By now you know that my mission (my "WHY") is to do everything in my power to create a positive legacy for my family. I truly hope you have made the decision to join me on this mission. If so, congratulations! There are thousands of us who have joined this team and we've all committed to creating a positive legacy for our own families. Please join us...more info is found on www.BuffMother.com.

However, I need to let you in on a little secret... None of us are even close to perfect! We all go through occasional slumps filled with bad choices. However, we are all very well educated in a very powerful law. The law that I'm referring to is the law of BuffMother! Momentum (BUFFMoJo). It's a little corny, but you'll never forget it! You need to be an expert in this law. The reason this law is so important is because it can be applied to every concept in this book.

"Every woman can create a legacy of health, fitness and success simply by creating positive momentum one tiny step at a time."

Train your Brain

Foundation #7: Massive Momentum!

Hormonal Timing is all about momentum down to its core. The pattern of Buffing, Boosting, Buffing, Boosting, etc, choreographed with your hormonal cycle creates MASSIVE MOMENTUM!! This is why we smash through plateaus so much easier than other women. Everything is spelled out, all you have to do is follow the program, use the tools, and you will automatically create massive momentum in your body, but what about your mind? Remember, the goal of this section is to Train Your Brain. The ingredients include Belief, Positive Mental Attitude, Energizing Others, a Legacy Perspective and the final ingredient to a BUFF BRAIN is Massive Momentum!

Break the negative pattern!

A minute ago I mentioned that nobody makes wise choices every time. However, you can be perfect in one area. You can be perfect in the art of breaking a negative momentum pattern. In other words, you never want to let negative momentum build. You must stop it dead in its tracks! Have you ever noticed that the longer you go without exercising, the tougher it is to MAKE yourself start up again? Personally, if I go more than 2 days without doing some sort of exercise, it takes a cattle prod to get me off my lazy butt!! The same goes for eating veggies, drinking my water, etc. I know that when I get into one of these negative momentum patterns, I must go back to the basics and take action immediately to get my BuffMoJo headed in the right direction. Momentum always fuels more momentum!

Every wise choice creates eternal benefits:

I believe that every positive choice you make concerning attitude, diet and fitness carries lifelong benefits. Simply put, every time you exercise, your body changes for the better on a cellular level. Nobody can take it away from you!! **I'm talking about: every set, rep, cardio session, vegetable you eat, glass of water you drink, etc. Every good decision affects every cell of your body in a positive way forever!** When you truly understand this fact, it is powerful!

You must focus all your energy on doing everything in your power to create massive momentum toward reaching your goal. The more momentum you create, the faster you will be successful!! Keep in mind that every tiny little thing has an effect on your momentum. If you aren't doing something to gain "MoJo" you're losing it!

I know this might sound a little intimidating so let's simplify. You must understand that success or failure will be determined by the **little things** that you do on a daily basis. You need to choose get healthy and fit! You get "buff", with every decision you make daily. If you make good choices, your momentum will continue to build and you will continually move in a positive direction. It's the little things that you do habitually and consistently that create massive momentum.

I call the LITTLE THINGS you do daily the "BuffMoJo Basics." They are guaranteed to get your momentum moving in a positive direction. By now, you know that I believe in keeping things simple. However, I almost never describe anything as "easy." The GREAT thing about the BuffMoJo Basics is that they are all simple and easy!! Use them when you are stuck in a negative momentum pattern.

The BuffMoJo Basics:
Drink a glass of water
Eat a green veggie
Exercise for 2 minutes
Write down a positive affirmation
Write down 5 things you are thankful for
Identify 3 positive qualities in the next person you see
Pay someone a genuine compliment
Encourage someone
Stand up and stretch
Take 5 deep breaths, exhaling completely after each one.
Clean something for 2 minutes
Stretch for 3 minutes
Eat a piece of fruit
Eat a carrot
Take your Hormonal Timing Pill and multivitamin.
Avoid the temptation to do something negative - this counts as doing something positive!

Let's use a mental illustration:

Picture a train parked on tracks that lead up a long gradual hill. This train represents your momentum. At the top of the hill is success, your dream, life goals, etc.). At the bottom of the hill is a bottomless pit called failure. Every positive imprint is fuel for the train making it speed up the hill. Every negative imprint is like lead weighing the train down. Remember, you are either gaining speed going up the hill, creating positive momentum to your goal, or you are rolling backwards towards destroying your momentum and possibly even creating a negative legacy.

Start making even little decisions based on whether or not it will create positive momentum or negative momentum toward your goals. Every positive thought, deed, comment, action, and choice has the power to create more momentum. You literally have thousands of opportunities every single day to gain momentum!!

Water or Coke?
Supplements over candy
Lettuce over cookies
Blueberries instead of ice cream
Banana over cereal bar

Oatmeal instead of fruit loops
Walk instead of a drive
Gym over mall
Workout vs. happy hour

Train your Brain

Success Tool #7- " 5 Minute MoJo"

You can regain and build Momentum in less than 5 minutes! Do the little things listed below to create instant positive momentum ~

"5 Minute MoJo"
1- drink 10 oz of water
2- march for 1 minute
3- take 5 full deep breaths
4- stretch for 1 minute
5- eat a green veggie!

"You have control over every decision! The big picture is made up of the little things!"

Let's review how all aspects of Training your Brain will allow you to create momentum and allow you to reach the "next level"! You can radically change your body, life and legacy using these foundational principles!!

1) **Believe**
- In order to accomplish your dreams, you MUST first believe with all your heart, soul and mind that you will succeed! To be blunt, if you don't believe, you are destined to fail!!
- Doubt kills belief.
- You must make a habit of crushing all doubt the second it pops into your mind.
- The best tool to crush doubt is a "truth hammer" (your positive affirmation).
- You must become a PRO at using your "truth hammer" to crush every doubt. Drill this into your brain.

2) **Positive Mental Attitude (PMA)**
- A PMA has the power to overcome any obstacle.
- A negative mental attitude is the result of constantly focusing on your problems.
- Negative mental attitudes are contagious.
- Don't spend time with anyone that has a NMA (negative mental attitude).
- The best way to create a PMA is to focus your energy on solutions.
- Focusing on Solutions will create hope.
- Hope is the only long-term fuel for a PMA

Train your Brain

3) Create Exponential Energy
- Motivation, Inspiration, Focus, Will, and Determination are all forms of energy.
- Every form of energy that you will need to accomplish your dreams is governed by The Law of Exponential Energy.
- You can tap into exponential energy if you're willing to pour your energy into helping others.
- Every time you release any form of positive energy or plant "energy seeds," energy will come back to you multiplied exponentially.
- The negative energy you pour out will flow back to you according to the same law.

4) Live with a Legacy Perspective
- If your "why" revolves solely around a measured visible result it is a "Weak Why"
- A "STRONG WHY" is critical for achieving big time success!! And, it must revolve around the people you love.
- Understand that your choices will leave eternal imprints on everything. These imprints will eventually become your Legacy.
- Foundation #6-Living your life with a "Legacy Perspective." This will result in success in other areas such as weight loss, more energy, etc...
- Success tool #6- the 24 Hour Legacy Test, really puts things in proper perspective.

5) Massive Momentum!
- Momentum is either positive or negative
- You must become a master at stopping negative momentum
- BuffMoJo Basics are the LITTLE THINGS you can do to gain positive momentum
- Success Tool # 7 "5 Minute MoJo" gives you a quick and easy strategy to stop a negative momentum pattern dead in it's tracks.

Now that you know why and how Hormonal Timing works and the importance of training your brain, you are set to take ACTION!

"Relentless motivation is achieved when a woman is motivated by the vision of each positive choice magnified a thousand times. When that vision drives every choice she makes, she cannot be stopped."

Train your Brain

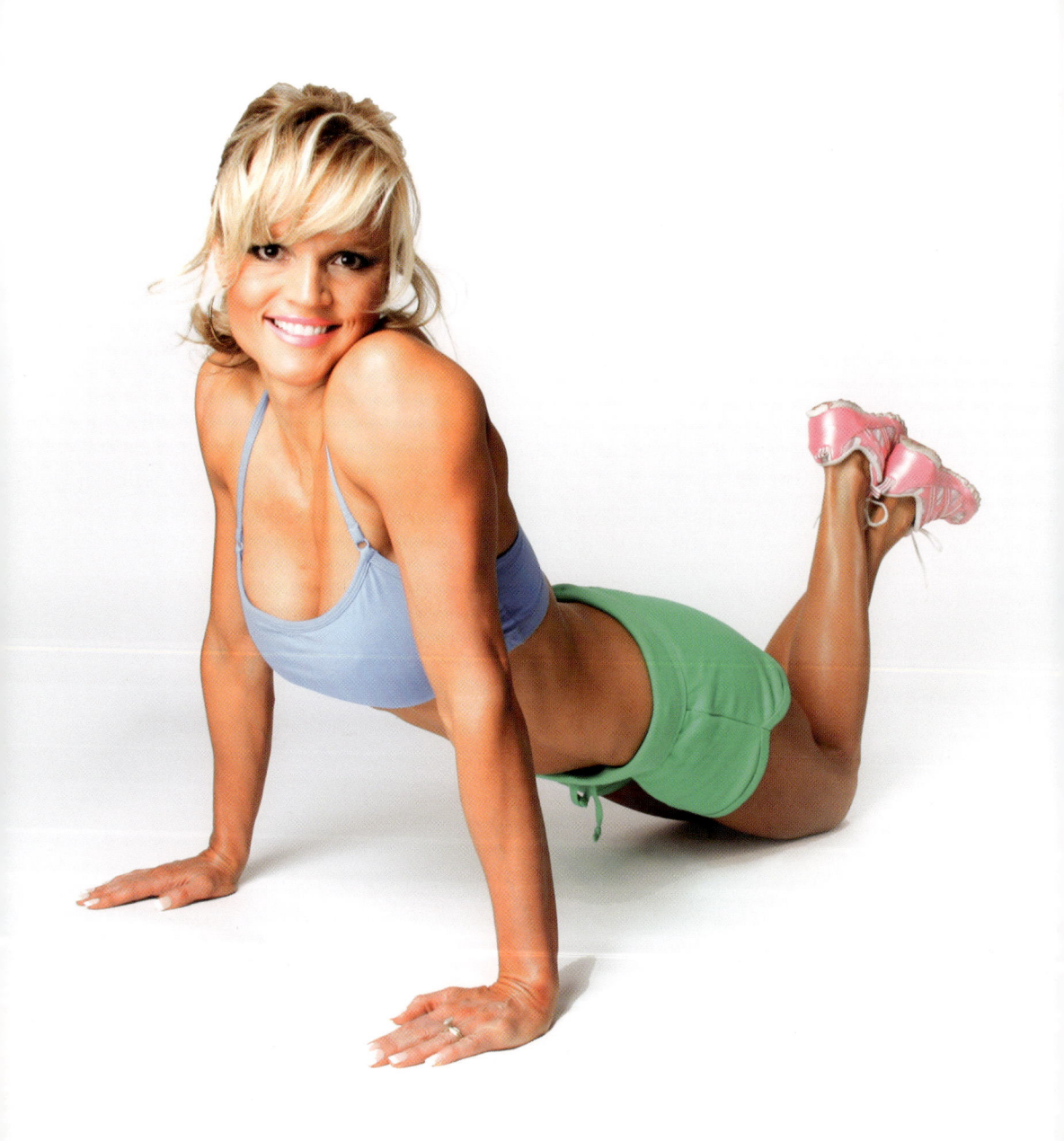

Nuts & Bolts for ACTION!

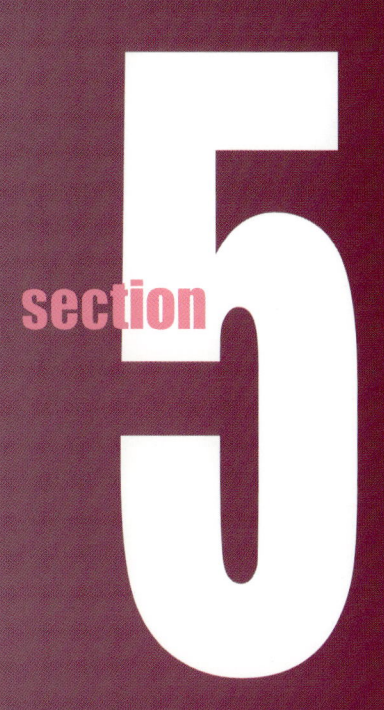

section 5

7 BuffMother! Fitness Truths:

1- You must consider your HORMONES!!

Of course, I have to have this on the TOP of the list! Hormonal Timing is a lifestyle. Without taking your hormones into consideration, you will be frustrated. By listening and responding to your body and utilizing the Buffing and Boosting phases, Hormonal Timing will produce results quicker and with more ease than you ever thought possible. Rest when you need rest, push when it is time to push, eat when you need to eat, etc...It is time to live life in TUNE with your natural biorhythms.

I have included a beginner workout program in this book. HOWEVER, I know every fitness program will become more effective when utilizing the foundations and success tools of Hormonal Timing. If you have a fitness plan you truly love, you can use the principles of Hormonal Timing to enhance it! This is what I call the OVERLAY philosophy of Hormonal Timing.

"Overlay Philosophy" of Hormonal Timing means you can use Hormonal Timing to ENHANCE the results of any diet and fitness program!!!

You can apply HT to any training program: running, resistance programs, women's gym programs, conditioning classes, DVDs, home gym machines, Pilates, etc. All you need to do is utilize all the FOUNDATIONS in this book along with applying the following KEYS to your favorite workouts according to what phase you are on in your cycle.

Apply these Buffing Keys:	Apply these Boosting Keys:
Have intense, high-quality workouts	Work out for a release; something is better than nothing
Maintain muscle mass while losing weight	Body is poised to build muscle, so use it!
Utilize the power of interval training	Any and all cardio is great, just get moving
Try to lose weight and progress in your fitness level	Maintenance of weight loss from Buffing- take a break from your caloric deficit and aim to maintain
Work out 4-6 days a week	Take an extra day of rest if needed; work out only 3-5 days per week
Take the Buffing Hormonal Timing Pill	Take Boosting Hormonal Timing Pill

2- If you want to be your BEST, Strength training is a MUST!!

Strength training increases metabolism.... Remember when you were young and able to eat whatever you wanted and not gain a pound? You had natural muscle tone and a much higher metabolism as a result! Strength training will enable you to re-build muscle on your body. AND, if you rebuild your body to where you have the muscles you did as a teen, you will once again successfully attain and maintain the body you desire. To have a strong metabolism you must have a good base of muscle on your body.

Other Great Benefits of Strength Training:
- An effective way to burn calories- not only during but up to 3 days afterward!
- Reverses and helps prevent signs of aging
- Strengthens your joints, ligaments and tendons
- Prevents injury
- Helps your balance and coordination
- Rebuilds bone density and prevents bone density loss
- Decreases risk of diabetes

Nuts and Bolts for ACTION

- Lowers resting blood pressure
- Elevates mood
- Increases the speed of digestion
- Increases HDL (good cholesterol)
- Lowers resting heart rate

3- Lifting will NOT make you bulky!

Ladies!!! The women you see that are bulky from lifting weights are often using illegal supplements (steroids, etc.) to get that way! As women, 95 percent or more of us do not have the natural ability to grow big muscles. The amount of testosterone in our bodies is 1/10th to 1/14th that of a man's. You just can't get bulky!

Instead, you will be building firmer, denser, healthier looking muscles. You will regain a youthful shape to your body. You will become more agile, bouncy, and controlled in your movements. Carrying in the groceries will be EASY. Loads of laundry won't be a danger to your back. You will be able to perform in life and look graceful at the same time!!

Youth Beauty vs. Buff Beauty

There are 2 kinds of beauty: Youth Beauty AND Buff Beauty. Youth beauty is mainly what we see in magazines, on TV and the internet. You don't need to work hard for beauty when you are young. It is just there. Think back to what your body looked and felt like in high school. What is the main difference between how it looks and feels now?

- Do you have a pouchy tummy where there once was a flat area?
- Do you have a saggy, uninspiring booty where there once was a cute little tooshie?
- Do you have the old lady "chicken wings" where you once had arms?

Guess what? Muscle tone is the key difference in your body now. Why do you think most models are between 18-24 with no kids? Did you know that the second you were done with puberty, you started losing muscle? That's why youth beauty fades with age. Muscle loss is accelerated by going through pregnancy, illness or periods of inactivity. In time your "body" will be gone unless you've done something to keep your muscle.

Women have chased "youth" beauty through aerobics, dieting, endless cardio, yoga, and many other non-muscle building strategies for years. You can chase youth beauty, but you will never catch it – you will only be left with a "skinny fat body" at best. In order to have an amazingly beautiful body again, you need to chase after the right kind of beauty, Buff Beauty™. Buff Beauty is found in a body rebuilt through regaining lost muscle mass, through consistent workouts and eating to perform in life. Muscle is what gives your body it's beautiful shape!

Nuts and Bolts for ACTION

4- Challenge yourself!

The diet industry has convinced us that our problem is that we need to lose weight. As a result, we spend billions on diet pills every year. "This new diet pill will help you lose 40 lbs in 3 weeks!! You'll look great in time for bikini season." Or, "You can have incredible ABS in 30 days simply by using this machine for 90 seconds a day!" These are LIES, and they lead to failure every time.

The only real way to change your body is to challenge it. Challenge= Change. When strength training use weights or resistance that challenges you. You need to challenge your muscles above and beyond what's easy to cause change! It is not EASY~ but it is 100 percent worth it. Trust me being buff is the BEST!!

Challenge=Change
Our bodies are master adapters. The more we challenge them the more they change to accommodate those demands. The good news about this is that if you continually challenge yourself, your body will change. The bad news is that if you **don't** continually challenge it, it will stop changing and may even regress.

There are 5 main ways to change workouts to cause them to be more challenging:

Intensity How hard are you pushing? Do you push yourself to the MAX each workout? Do you only ever "go through the motions"—social exerciser? Do you vary your intensity to get different results? Do you like to take your time? Do you like to "get it done"?

Frequency How often do you work out? How often do you lift each body part? How often do you do intervals? How often do you do other fitness activities?

Duration How long do you workout at a time? How long are your lifting sessions? How long are your intervals? How much other time do you devote to fitness activities?

Mode What type of activities do you do? Do you cross train? Are you training for a certain sport? What lifts do you do for each body part?

Rest intervals How many "rest" days do you take? How much time between each lifting set/exercise do you do? How much time between hard intervals do you "rest"? How much time do you "rest" each day? Do you purposely take time to "de-stress"?

Nuts and Bolts for ACTION

5- Quality over Quantity

You DO NOT have to spend much time working out to get results. If you work hard, even 10 minutes can make a big impact. HOURS of cardio are often a waste of time. Choose the most effective exercises and PUSH your body. Focus on your BIG MUSCLES (Legs, Back and Chest) and on using BIG MOVEMENTS. If you focus on HIGH quality exercise and keep active in life, you don't need much quantity.

6- TIME!!

It takes time to see results from any exercise program. I have asked many of my clients, "how many years of abuse are you trying to erase?" Often times the answer is 10 years or more. I then ask "Why do you think you can erase 10 years in 10 weeks?" It is not possible. It will take time!! But you CAN do it, in TIME! The greatest thing about strength training is that it is <u>cumulative</u> when done consistently. Each workout builds upon the last and in time your results will blow you away. If you consistently lift 2-3 times per week you will see continual change. You will get stronger, more coordinated, more flexible, in better shape and feel tighter!! TIME is CRUCIAL.

7- Fuel your body to perform. Your body needs nutrients!!

This subject hits the very heart of my philosophy! What are your goals when you go to the gym? Do you want to have a good, enjoyable workout that causes residual effects by increasing your fitness level and your overall health and happiness? OR do you want to squeeze every tiny little milligram of possible fat burning out of your hour of hellacious cardio so that you can try to do the same thing again day, after day, after day, after day…?

The general rule is to have a small meal with carbs and protein 1.5 to 2 hours before your workout. Oatmeal and a small chicken breast is a great choice. Please see the diet and supplementation chapter for more information on how to incorporate eating to perform into your lifestyle. Please remember the long-term goal is to rebuild youthful muscle that will burn the fat off your body!

"The path of least resistance leads to a poor reflection in the mirror."

Foundation #8: Plan of Attack! (POA)

How to TAKE ACTION and DO IT NOW!!

Now that you know how to track your cycle and have a good knowledge base about how the Buffing and Boosting phases work, it's time to make your Plan of Attack of POA to apply Hormonal Timing to your personal fitness and diet program:

On this chart you see the Buffing days in PINK and Boosting days in PURPLE. If you have an average 28-day monthly cycle, your Buffing and Boosting phases will be exactly 2 weeks each. The Buffing Phase runs from c-day 5 through c-day 18. The Boosting phase runs from c-day 19 through c-day 28 and then continues on from c-day 1 to c-day 4. On a chart like this or on a normal calendar, you need to note when you will be in your Buffing and Boosting Phases. As I have shown in this example:

Buffing Phase

	MON	TUE	WED	THU	FRI	SAT	SUN
Week 1	c-day 5 June 6	c-day 6	c-day 7	c-day 8	c-day 9	c-day 10	c-day 11
Week 2	c-day 12	c-day 13	c-day 14	c-day 15	c-day 16	c-day 17	c-day 18 June 19

Boosting Phase

	MON	TUE	WED	THU	FRI	SAT	SUN
Week 3	c-day 19 June 20	c-day 20	c-day 21	c-day 22	c-day 23	c-day 24	c-day 25
Week 4	c-day 26	c-day 27	c-day 28	c-day 1	c-day 2	c-day 3	c-day 4 July 3

Make a mental note, *"I will be Buffing starting June 6th through June 19th"*...Then after those 2 weeks note, *"I will be Boosting starting June 20th through July 3rd."*

Nuts and Bolts for ACTION

RULE
When in doubt BUFF (i.e. add days to your Buffing phase)

Rule Examples:
- If your cycle runs longer than 28 days add additional days to Buffing. For instance, if you have a 30-day cycle you will need to add 2 days to Buffing. You will be Buffing for 16 days and Boosting for 14 days.
- If your cycle runs short, subtract days from Boosting. For instance, if you have a 26-day cycle you need to subtract 2 days of Boosting. You will be Buffing for 14 days and Boosting for 12 days.
- If you have irregular cycles, go by the last month's cycle length to figure the next month's phases, unless you see an every other month pattern. Our ovaries typically take turns and one may cause a shorter cycle while the other may cause a longer cycle.

Keep this chart handy to help you REMEMBER to apply the KEYS to Successful Buffing and Boosting.

Buffing c-day 5-18	Boosting c-day 19-28 and 1-4
Be relentless - Give it 110%	Rest a bit more - slow the pace
Think, "I can do anything for 2 weeks!"	Realize, "It's just my hormones."
Focus on weight loss and diet - caloric deficit	Boost your metabolism - eat to fuel your workouts
Eat CLEAN to lose weight	Maintain weight loss
Do extra activities and cardio	Cut back on workout frequency or duration
Buff your body - BODYBuffing	
Take Buffing Hormonal Timing Pill	Focus on doing "something"
	Take Boosting Hormonal Timing Pill

Before you Begin...
General Training Rules:
1. Make sure to warm up for 5-10 minutes before your lifting workout. Something simple like walking or the recumbent bike works well. You will perform better and prevent injury if you are "warm" and have your blood pumping.
2. At this point you need to try to do your lifting before cardio/intervals. You need to use the bulk of your energy for your lifting.
3. Make sure to do at least a few ab exercises every time you workout. Be sure to continually be conscious of your form and posture 24/7 including during your workouts.
4. Make sure to keep a workout log so that you can track your progress- use the Foundations Success Journal, a notebook or a blog.

5. On leg day, try not to do much cardio or intervals; the leg workout will be draining enough.

Detailed strength training instructions:
1- <u>Challenge yourself on each lift</u>
- Use the first set as a warm-up, focusing on proper form and breathing and making sure to think about the muscles you are working.
- Second set: Increase the weight used to where the last 2 reps are very hard
- Third set: Continue to challenge yourself and increase the weight if needed to where you can barley do the last 2 reps.

2- <u>Recovery between sets</u>
- During the Beginner Buffing phase, have little or no rest between exercises.
- During the Beginner Boosting phase rest one minute between sets (stretching is great to do during your "rest").

3- <u>Remember to breathe</u>
- This is VITAL!! Your muscles need oxygen to work.
- Exhale on the exertion (contraction)
- Inhale on the lowering or stretching motion (eccentric)

4- <u>Controlled Movements</u>
- For your pace, use a 3/2 count. (detailed below)
- The concentric (lifting/effort motion) 2 counts (1-2).
- Pause, hold and squeeze at the end of the concentric motion
- The eccentric motion (easy motion/lowering of weight) should take 3 counts (1-2-3)

What you can expect:
- You will get sore at first! Please know that after the initial set of workouts your soreness will be the worst. If you are consistent, your soreness will not be as intense.
- Make sure to eat enough protein and drink tons of water. This will help the soreness dissipate.
- You will get stronger very quickly, so make sure to always try to up the weights (remember challenge=change). You will have a big initial strength increase due to your mind/body connecting to perform the movement. Once your brain "connects" with your body your strength will "spike"!
- You will have some small aches and pains. You are rebuilding muscles, tendons, ligaments and bones, so don't be surprised if they get a little "sore." Please, listen to your body and make sure to ease off if something really hurts.

Success Tool #8: Step-by-Step Illustrated Exercise Plan

Includes a detailed workout calendar, strength training routine and cardio-vascular fitness program.

Beginner Buffing Phase workout calendar

	MON	TUE	WED	THU	FRI	SAT	SUN
Week 1	c-day 5 Lift upper body	c-day 6 Intervals*	c-day 7 Lift lower body	c-day 8 Active Rest -i.e. housework or shop	c-day 9 Lift upper body	c-day 10 Intervals	c-day 11 off
Week 2	c-day 12 Lift lower body	c-day 13 Intervals	c-day 14 Lift upper body	c-day 15 Active Rest -i.e. housework or shop	c-day 16 Lift lower body	c-day 17 Intervals	c-day 18 off

*See page 93 for intervals info and instructions

Summary of Beginner Buffing Phase:
- 3 lifting workouts per week
- Workout is a circuit: do exercises in order a total of 3 times
- Very little rest between exercises
- 2 interval sessions and 1 active rest day each week
- Focus on dieting and losing weight

Buffing Reminder Chart

Be relentless- give it 110%
Think, "I can do anything for 2 weeks!"
Focus on weight loss and diet- caloric deficit
Eat CLEAN to lose weight
Do extra activities and cardio
Buff your body- BODY Buffing
Be aware of your Ovulation
Take The Hormonal Timing Pill (pink) Buffing Pill daily

Nuts and Bolts for ACTION

Beginner Buffing - Upper body Circuit

Do the following 8 exercises in the order listed, **complete the entire list 3 times.**

1. Push Ups on Knees- 10 repetitions

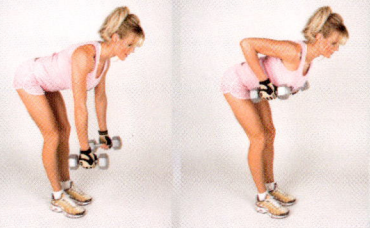

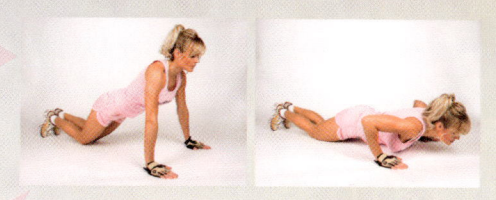

2. Bent over DB rows- 10 repetitions

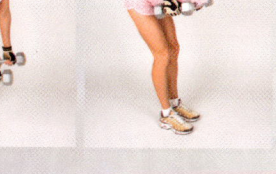

3. Chair Dips- 10 repetitions

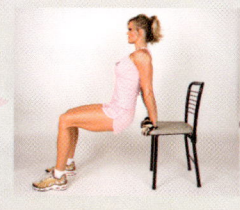

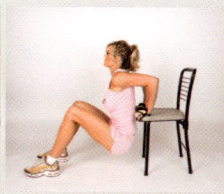

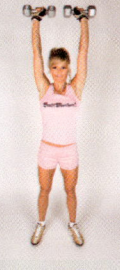

4. Shoulder press- 10 repetitions

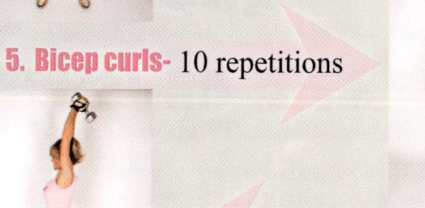

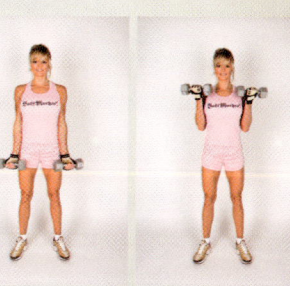

5. Bicep curls- 10 repetitions

6. Tricep extensions- 10 repetitions

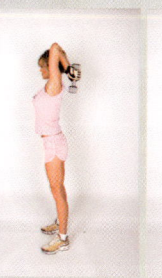

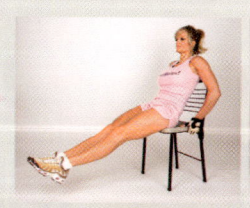

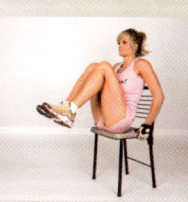

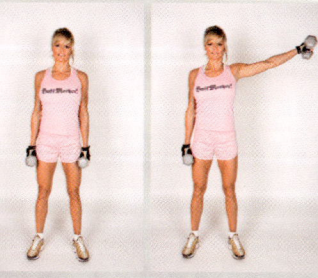

7. Ab Knee ups- 15 repetitions

8. Lateral shoulder raises- alternate arms, 10 repetitions each

Nuts and Bolts for ACTION

Beginner Buffing-Lower Body Circuit

Do the following 7 exercises in the order listed, **complete the entire list 3 times.**
* Start with no weight on these exercises

1. DB Squats*- 15 repetitions

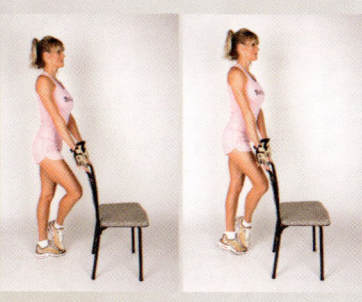

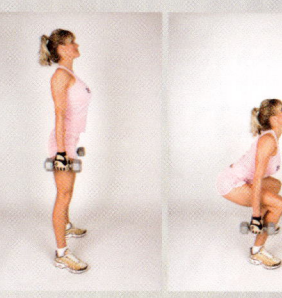

2. Calf Raises- 10 repetitions

3. Stationary Lunges*- 10 repetitions

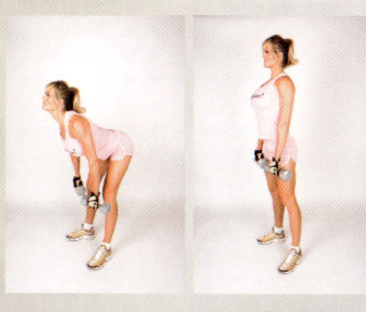

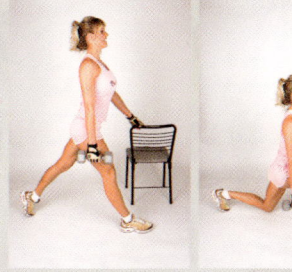

4. Dead lifts- 15 repetitions

4. Crunches- 15 repetitions

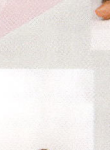

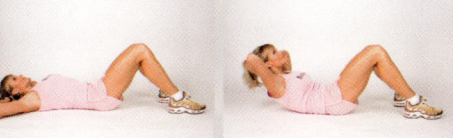

6. Side leg lifts- 15 repetitions

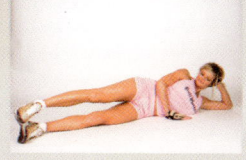

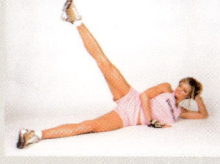

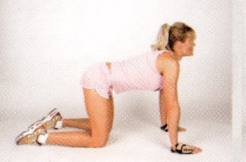

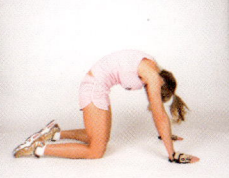

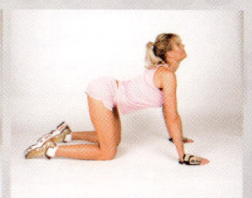

7. CATS -n -DOGS
Hold each position for four seconds. Repeat four times.

Nuts and Bolts for ACTION

Beginner Boosting Phase Workout Calendar

	MON	TUE	WED	THU	FRI	SAT	SUN
Week 3	c-day 19 Lift upper body	c-day 20 Intervals	c-day 21 Lift lower body	c-day 22 Active Rest -i.e. housework or shop	c-day 23 Lift upper body	c-day 24 Intervals	c-day 25 off
Week 4	c-day 26 Lift lower body	c-day 27 Intervals	c-day 28 Lift upper body	c-day 1 Active Rest -i.e. housework or shop	c-day 2 Lift lower body	c-day 3 Intervals	c-day 4 off

Summary of Beginner Boosting Phase:

- 3 lifting workouts per week
- 3 sets of 10 traditional style lifting- do all sets of one exercise before moving to the next
- 1 min rest period between sets of each exercise
- 2 interval sessions post lifting or non-lifting days
- Focus on resting a bit more and getting stronger!

Boosting Reminder Chart

Rest a bit more- slow the pace
Realize, "It's just my hormones"
Boost your metabolism- eat to fuel your workouts
Maintain your weight loss
Cut back on workout frequency or duration
Focus on doing "something"; strength training is extra productive
You're hungrier because you need more food
Take The Hormonal Timing Pill (purple) Boosting Pill daily

Nuts and Bolts for ACTION

Beginner Boosting - Upper body training

Complete 3 sets of each exercise then move to the next listed, **allow 1 min rest between each set.**

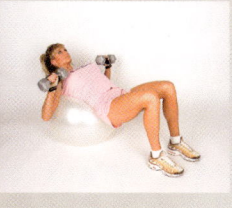

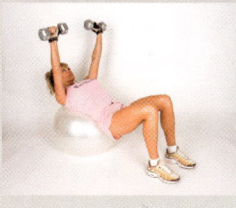

1. DB Chest press- 3 sets of 10 repetitions (3x10) on ball or bench

2. Push ups on Knees- 3 sets of 10 (3x10)

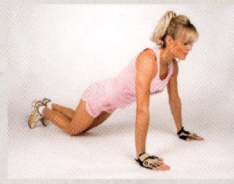

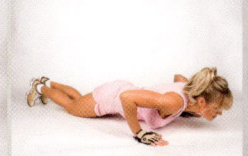

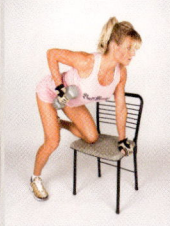

3. One arm bent over Lat rows- 3 sets of 10 (3x10)

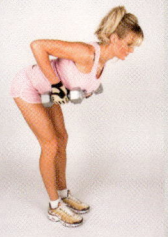

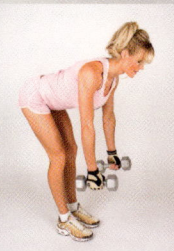

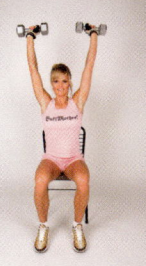

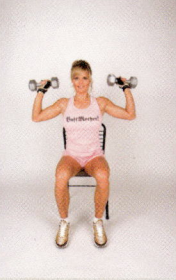

4. Bent over DB rows- 3 sets of 10 (3x10)

5. Shoulder Press- 3 sets of 10 (3x10)

6. Bicep Curls- 3 sets of 10 (3x10)

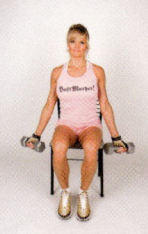

7. Chair Dips- 3 sets of 10 (3x10)

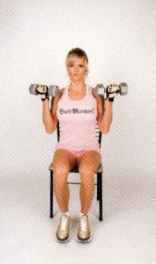

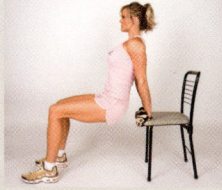

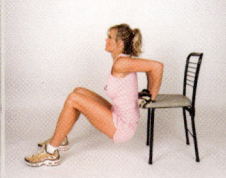

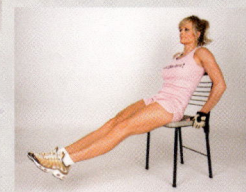

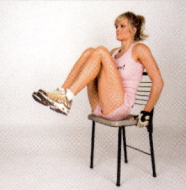

8. Ab knee ups- 3 sets of 15 (3x15)

Nuts and Bolts for ACTION

Beginner Boosting-Lower Body Training

Complete 3 sets of each exercise then move to the next listed, **allow 1 min rest between each set.**

1. **DB Squats-** 3 sets of 10 repetitions (3x10)

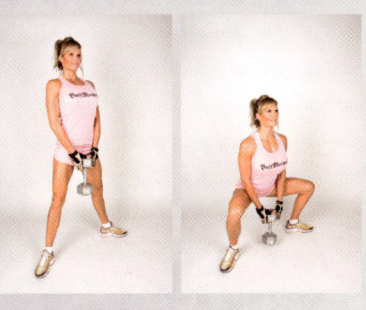

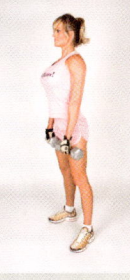

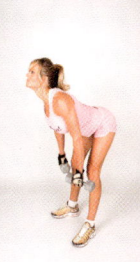

2. **Plies Squats-** 3 sets of 10 (3x10)

3. **Dead lifts-** 3 sets of 10 (3x10)

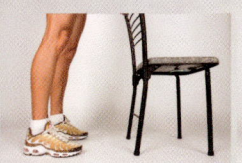

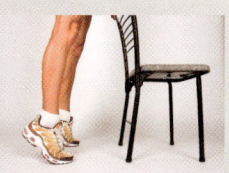

4. **Calf raises-** 3 sets of 10 (3x10)

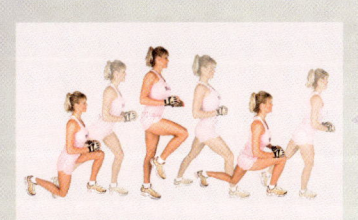

5. **Ball leg curls-** 3 sets of 15 (3x15)

6. **Walking Lunges-** 3 sets of 10 each leg (3x10)

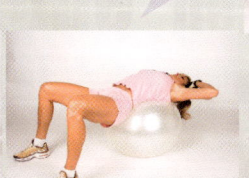

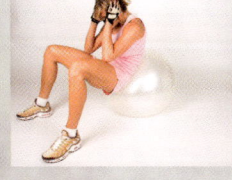

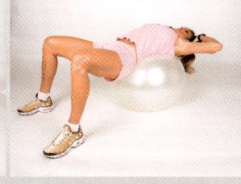

7. **Ab/Adductors or "V's"-** 3 sets of 15 (3x15)

8. **Ball Crunches-** 3 sets of 15 (3x15)

Nuts and Bolts for ACTION

"BuffMotherobics!"™: Intervals

I recommend doing most cardio in the form of interval training. I call my intervals "BuffMotherobics!" A simple 20-minute "BuffMotherobics!" interval workout will provide optimal results in minimal time. It's perfect for those of us who have no time or desire to spend hours doing cardio.

Science has proven that interval training gives the following results:

1. INCREASES FITNESS- Interval training increases overall fitness (both Aerobic and Anaerobic capacity) and efficiency of cardiac and lung function.

2. BURNS CALORIES- Interval training increases energy production (increased metabolic rate) for up to 72 hours after a single session.

3. BURNS FAT- Interval training increases your body's efficiency of using fat for fuel (you will burn the fat off your butt and gut!)

4. INCREASE CONTRACTION- Interval training increases ability of muscle contraction (great news for being able to build a great metabolism and move with controlled ease).

5. BOOSTS BRAIN FUNCTION- Interval training causes an increase in mental sharpness and clarity.

Interval Training "BuffMotherobics!"	VS. Cardio - low intensity steady aerobics
Stimulating and Quick (20 min.)	Boring and Lengthy (45-60 min.)
In the long term and short term increases your metabolism (Anabolic "Building up")	In the long term decreases metabolism (Catabolic "Tearing down")
Energizing- increases energy output for up to 48 hours	Energy Drain - uses up your extra energy stores
Less wear and tear on joints and muscles due to shorter duration and less volume	Leads to wear and tear on joints and muscles resulting in injuries
Increases muscle building/sparing hormone levels following session	Does not raise muscle building hormone levels
The best method for lowering body fat	Not the best method of lowering your body fat

Nuts and Bolts for ACTION

I choose intense **BuffMotherobics!** over traditional cardio for the following reasons:

- **Time-** I am busy and don't feel I can commit more than 20 mins to my cardio.
- **Results-** I get better and faster results from a focused, 20-min session of BuffMotherobics! than traditional long duration steady cardio. It energizes me versus draining me.
- **Fun factor-** time goes by faster when I play "games" with myself during my session. Moving from one speed to another often adds a dimension that keeps me from being bored.
- **Injury Prevention-** I have had "overuse" injuries and joint pain in the past from running too far, too long and too often. POUNDING adds up on joints. I like intervals because in 20 mins only so much pounding can happen and I can get great results with as little as 3 sessions a week. It is short and sweet, allowing my joints to rest the other 23 hours and 40 mins of the day.

Beginner BuffMotherobics!™ Interval Training
20 min is always the goal:
- 5 min. warm up
- 1 min. hard (i.e. walk fast)
- 2 min. easy (i.e. medium paced walk)
- 1 min. hard
- 2 min. easy
- 1 min. hard
- 2 min. easy
- 1 min. hard
- 5 min. cool down

This is 20 minutes total: 4 hard minutes total

*If you don't feel exhausted by the end, increase the intensity of all hard and/or easy minutes.

"I am on a mission to show every busy woman that the Hormonal Timing lifestyle is the shortest distance between who you are, and who you want to become!"

Foundation #9: Simple Diet and Supplementation

Let's start with a quick "refresher" course on some basic nutrition knowledge. There are 3 main macro-nutrients in food: Protein, Carbs and Fats. Let's explore the basic facts about these 3 macro-nutrients.

Protein:
- Protein has 4 calories per gram.
- Protein takes extra energy to digest, up to 1 calorie per gram. (so there is a net 3 calories per gram in protein).
- The most popular proteins are animal, milk-based, or soy-based.
- They require a lot of energy to be converted into body fat.
- Protein is essential for muscle maintenance and growth. They are the building blocks for your body.
- They can be converted to use for energy.
- They take up to 3 hours to digest.

Carbohydrates:
- Carbohydrates have 4 calories per gram.
- There are 2 types: simple (sugars) and complex (high fiber/nutrient dense).
- They are essential for quick energy.
- They are easily digested.
- They are easily converted into energy and easily converted into body fat.
- They are everywhere and they are sweet and/or salty and yummy.
- They are addictive and easily overeaten.
- They take as little as 10 mins or up to 2 hours to be digested.

Fats:
- Fats have 9 calories per gram.
- Fats are essential for proper brain and body function.
- They are vital to balanced hormone production.
- They are popularly broken into two categories: "good fats" (natural) and "bad fats" (man-altered).
- They are your muscle's primary source of energy.
- In excess, they are easily converted into body fat.
- They take up to 4 hours to be digested.

I am sick of traditional diets! Why have we convinced ourselves eating has to be complicated, unnatural or painful in order for our diet to work? My philosophy towards my diet is to KISS!! Apply KISS to your diet so you can do it for life! KISS stands for Keep It Simple Sweetheart. I DO NOT let myself be obsessed. Obsessive dieting does not work for life! You want to keep your diet simple enough to be a **lifestyle** not a kamikaze mission!

Nuts and Bolts for ACTION

Success Tool #9: The "5-4-3-2-1 Diet"*

THE goal is to consume the following number of portions daily:**

5- Protein (P)
Portions of approximately 25g each (palm size)

4-Carbohydrate (C)
Portions of approximately 25g each (fist size)

3- Fat (F) servings
Portions of approximately your goal weight in calories

2 to 3- Greens (G)
Big portions (one cup minimum)- fill up with greens.

1 Optional Treat (T)
Portions of approximately your goal weight in calories

11 -(10 oz.) Water (W)
Portions minimum

*Instructions for "Buffing" Diet:
OMIT one carb/day (add more greens)
OMIT treat
So for portions during Buffing: 5P-3C-3F-3G

**PORTION INFO

General portion sizes are based on a woman working out 4 times a week with the goal of losing weight and fat, and **goal weight** between 115-135 pounds. For alternate goal weight ranges use these portions for Proteins and Carbohydrates:

Under 115#= about 20g portion sizes
115-135= about 25g portion sizes
Over 136# = about 30g portion sizes

- Fat and Treat portions sizes= your <u>goal</u> weight in calories.
- GREENS are unlimited in portion sizes (at least 1cup), so eat up!!
- Water= any non-caffeinated, non-sugared drink can count as water. Drink a minimum of 11 portions daily.

<u>DISCLAIMER:</u> Portion sizes and caloric ranges vary widely based on a variety of factors (body composition, age, fitness history, health history, genetics, activity level, personality, etc.). There is no one size fits all portion size or caloric intake. Please, keep in mind this is just a "general" guide.

<u>Nuts and Bolts for ACTION</u>

To measure portions, try to use the EASIEST method most often:
1. My general rule is to go by the palm/fist eyeball method of keeping portions in check. For your proteins serving choose a portion the size of your palm and for carbs eat an amount equal to the size of your fist.
2. Reading labels comes in very handy in determining portion sizes for many foods.
3. You can also weigh your food with a food scale, if you feel you need a more exact measurement. Personally, I have never used a scale (besides to try it out). *NOTE- Keep in mind that each ounce of meat typically contains about 6g of protein (1oz meat=6g protein)

Simply chart your portions:

As you go through your day, keep track of what you've eaten. The most important components are **Protein**, **Greens** and **Water**. Focus on these the most. If you are ever truly hungry, after having all of your allotted servings for the day, you can have additional proteins or greens.

Simple ways to chart include:
1. Use a notebook or whiteboard and write P for protein, C for carb, F for Fat, G for Greens, T for treat, and W for Water as you go through your day.
2. Use a cross off chart like this (included in your success journal log):

DATE: _____ (Boosting)　　　　DATE: _____ (Buffing)
Daily Eating Record　　　　　　**Daily Eating Record**
P P P P P　　　　　　　　　　　　P P P P P
C C C C　　　　　　　　　　　　　C C C C
F F F　　　　　　　　　　　　　　F F F
G G __　　　　　　　　　　　　　 G G __
T　　　　　　　　　　　　　　　　T
W W W W W W W W W W　　　　　　W W W W W W W W W W
Notes: _____　Notes: _____
_____　_____

"The KEY to a successful diet is to make it a LIFESTYLE."

Nuts and Bolts for ACTION

97

When choosing your foods, keep a few things in mind:

- Choose natural foods over man-made foods (artificial sweeteners, low fat products, packaged/processed foods, etc). I would rather see you eat "whole fat" items than man-made toxins. They are not worth using to "save" calories. Instead of helping your weight loss efforts, they will leave you with toxins in your body. Toxins create all sorts of issues ranging from bloating, muscle aches, digestive issues, swollen glands, cellulite, skin blemishes, etc. Try your best to eliminate them from your diet. FLUSH those toxins out!! This is termed eating "CLEAN."
- I highly encourage you to vary your food choices. For instance, my daily goal for my protein intake is to have one portion of red meat, one of eggs, one of poultry, one of fish, and one of soy or whey. Variety is needed both for you mentally and physically. The same thing goes for your carbohydrate, fat and green choices.
- Try to limit your protein supplements (powders, bars, etc.) to 1 (at most 2) servings a day- real food is always best.

Expect a Learning Curve toward LIFESTYLE!!

The key to a successful diet is to make it a LIFESTYLE. As I mentioned earlier, KISS (Keep It Simple Sweetheart) is the best way to do this. My main focus on my diet is to keep it simple and doable with my crazy schedule. I now simply count my portions as I go through the day. However, when I first was learning to eat right, planning was a vital part of the learning curve. So get out your journal and PLAN how you can fit in the proper portions of your diet in each day. Soon you will be KISSing~

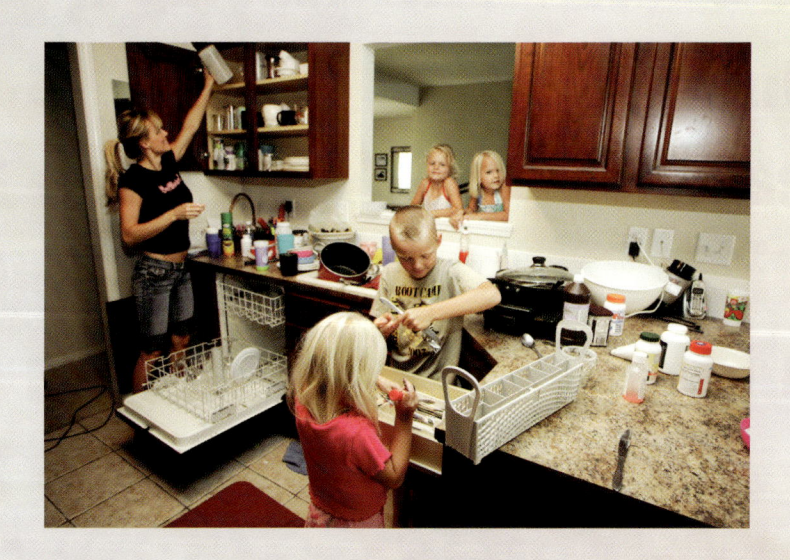

HOW To KISS:

#1- Plan to Perform
As I mentioned in "Fuel your body to perform," on page 83, timing your main carbohydrate (C) portions around workouts will allow you to have strong, effective and productive workouts.

#2- Proteins and greens
Fill up the rest of your daily meals with proteins (P) and greens (G) <u>then</u> your left over serving(s) of carbs (C).

#3- Work with your body
Make sure to account for your natural body rhythms. Are you a big morning eater or the opposite? I am a big evening eater, so I plan for that. I eat light in the morning and early afternoon because I know I'll easily get in the rest of my calories later. Don't ignore your natural tendencies if you want this to become a lifestyle vs. a short-term DIET.

#4- Eat often
Shoot to eat every 3-4 hours in order to keep an even energy flow. Remember the fact that food is FUEL...your body and mind don't function well on empty. Shoot for 4-5 meals daily.

#5- Fat can be GOOD
Make sure you are eating enough fat or you will be HUNGRY and be more tempted to cheat. Fat is also very important for proper hormone production, prevention of aging and maintenance of energy levels.

#6- Drink water like a fish!
Are you unsatisfied after a meal? Are you a bottomless pit? Oftentimes we feel this way when we are actually thirsty. Water is also an important transporter of both nutrients and toxins. Without enough, it is hard for your body to lose fat. So drink up! To optimize digestion, try to limit water consumption during your meals. Your main water consumption needs to be <u>between</u> meals, optimally 30 minutes prior and 30 minutes after meals.

Nuts and Bolts for ACTION

Handy Food lists to help you eat a variety of portion choices:

Proteins

Best Choice	Good Choice	To "get by" choice
Turkey	Other fish	Fried chicken strips
Chicken breasts	Shell fish	Fried fish
Steak, Roast, Brisket	Beef jerky	Pre-made hamburgers
Salmon	Turkey jerky	Fast Food meat
Tuna	Ham	Salami
Halibut	Lean Deli meat	Hot Dogs
Bass	Pre-cooked frozen meat	Protein bars
Flounder	Dark Poultry meat	Ready-to-drink protein
Haddock	Cottage cheese	Pork ribs
Eggs	Yogurt (sugar-free no flavor)	Cheese
Protein powders (pure)	Soy Milk (both a P and a C)	
Ground beef	Canned Sardines	
Ground poultry	Boca Burgers	
Tofu and Soy products	Other Protein powders	
Lean pork		

Carbohydrates

Best Choice	Good Choice	To "get by" choice
Oatmeal	Corn	Juice (fruit or veggie)
Barley	Grapes	Gatorade
Brown rice	Oranges	Cereal bars
Wild rice	Pears	Cereal
Sweet potato	Other fruit	Pancakes
Yam	Dried fruit	Bread
Squash	Potato (white)	Pasta
Beans	Whole wheat bread	Cake
Blueberries	White rice	Muffins
Strawberries	Whole wheat pasta	Crackers
Apple	Rice cakes	Other Yogurts (than sugar-free, no flavor)
Other berries	Milk (both a P and a C)	
Carrots		
Whole Grain cereal		
Chickpeas		
Kidney beans		
Ezekiel Bread		
Soy Milk (both a P and a C)		

Nuts and Bolts for ACTION

Fats

Best Choice	Limited Choice	To Eliminate
Fish oil	Vegetable oil	Hydrogenated fats
Olive oil	Other nuts	Fats in processes foods
Safflower oil	Peanut butter	Excessive saturated fats
Flax seed oil	Salad dressings	Margarine
Walnut oil	Cheeses	Fake butters
almonds	Cream cheese	No-fat cheese
Walnuts	Cream or half & half	No-fat dressings
Butter		
Cream		
Cashews (raw)		
Pistachios (raw, insides only)		
Olives		
Avocado		
Almond butter		
Coconut		
Peanut Butter (natural)		
Soy Butter		
Egg Yolks		

Greens (water-based or fibrous vegetables)

GREAT Choice	GREAT Choice	GREAT Choice
Alfalfa Sprouts	Collard Greens	Radishes
Artichoke Hearts	Cucumber	Rhubarb
Asparagus	Dandelion Greens	Sauerkraut
Bamboo Shoots	Eggplant	Scallions
Bean Sprouts	Fennel	Snow Pea Pods
Beet Greens	Hearts of Palm	Spaghetti Squash
Bock Choy	Kale	Spinach
Broccoli	Kohlrabi	String beans
Brussels Sprouts	Leeks	Summer Squash
Cabbage	Lettuce	Turnips
Cauliflower	Mushrooms	Tomatoes
Celery	Okra	Water Chestnuts
Celery Root	Onion	Wax beans
Chard	Parsley	Zucchini
Chicory	Peppers	Most SALSA
Chives	Pumpkin	

Treats
You don't need a list, do you? ☐

Nuts and Bolts for ACTION

The 5 - 4 - 3 - 2 - 1 Diet: Examples for Buffing and Boosting days based on workout times.

Buffing Days:
Total = 5P-3C-3F-3G

workout early AM	workout early PM	workout late PM
5:00am Preworkout Fasted cardio or if lifting Juice or fruit (banana) C	Extended fast - Maybe do some Fasted cardio?	Extended fast - Maybe do some Fasted cardio?
5:30am Workout	9:00am Meal 1: P C	8:00am-9:00am Meal 1: P G
7:00am Meal 1: P C	12:00pm Meal 2 (lunch): P C G F	11:00am-12:00pm Meal 2 (snack): P F G
10:00am Meal 2 (snack): P F	2:00pm Workout	2:00pm Meal 3 (lunch): P C F
2:00pm Meal 3 (lunch): P C F 2G	4:00pm Post Workout Meal 3: P C	5:00pm Pre-workout Meal 4: P C F G
6:00 Meal 4 (supper): 2P C(if none at 5am) F G	7:00pm Meal 4: 2P F 2G	7:00pm Workout
Extended fast - Evening Snack herbal tea	Evening Snack herbal tea	8:00pm-9:00pm Post Workout Meal Meal 5: P C
ALL Day/Night WATER!!	ALL Day/Night WATER!!	ALL Day/Night WATER!!

Nuts and Bolts for ACTION

Boosting Days:
Total = 5P-4C-3F-3G-T

workout early AM	workout early PM	workout late PM
5:00am Preworkout snack Juice or fruit (banana) C	8:00am Meal 1: P C T (a yummy coffee?)	8:00am Meal 1: P C
5:30am Workout	11:00am-12:00pm Pre-workout Meal 2 (lunch): P C G F	11:00am-12:00pm Meal 2 (snack): P F G
7:00am Postworkout Meal 1: Shake P C	2:00pm Workout	2:00pm Meal 3 (lunch): P C F T
10:00am Meal 2 (snack): snack P F	3:00pm-4:00pm Post workout Meal 3: C P	5:00pm Pre-workout Meal 4: P C F G
1:00pm-2:00pm Meal 3 (lunch): P C F G	7:00pm Meal 4 (supper): 2P C F G	7:00pm Workout
5:00pm-6:00pm (supper): Meal 4: P C F G		8:00pm-9:00pm Post workout Meal 5: P C
8:00pm Meal 5: P T		
ALL Day/Night WATER!!	ALL Day/Night WATER!!	ALL Day/Night WATER!!

Nuts and Bolts for ACTION

Let's talk about SUPPLEMENTATION!!

Why ordinary nutrition is not enough:
1. "Junk" food- Americans' diets are filled with fast food, processed foods, preserved foods, high-sugar and high-fat food.
2. Stimulants are being used in excess and interfere with proper food intake and nutrient absorption.
3. Less nutritious foods- farming methods (pesticides, hormones and fertilizers) have decreased the nutrient content in our foods.
4. Food processing- since food is imported from many places, methods are used to ensure a longer shelf life...all of which negatively impact nutrient content.
5. Dieting for weight loss- half of Americans are on a diet.
6. Stress- Environmental (chemicals, pollutants, hormones, pesticides, chlorine, plastic) all burden the liver to detoxify, which uses essential nutrients. Emotional and life stress also deplete nutrients and suppress the immune system

Supplementation 101

Over the past few years I've experimented with virtually every kind of legal lotion, potion, pill, etc. I recommend specific products to my private clients and make sure they "steer clear" of others. The bottom line: Some supplements are worth every penny while others are a waste of money.

Start with a good base of nutrients by taking:

A Multivitamin-
- A good multi is a must because of all the reasons listed above....our diets are never perfect enough.
- Make sure you find one that is time-released. If not, you may experience nausea due to everything hitting your system at in one big shot.
- Make sure it has been produced by a quality company. Quality is important.

Calcium-
- Vital for your bone and tooth health, proper muscle function and metabolism.
- Key for proper muscle and blood vessel contraction
- Needed for secretion of hormones

AND Take...
The Hormonal Timing Pill

As you can imagine, I highly recommend taking the Hormonal Timing (HT) Pill on a daily basis. Women have completely different nutrient needs at the beginning of the month vs. the end of the month. The Buffing and Boosting formulations of the Hormonal Timing Pill are designed to complement your body chemistry and goals as you progress through your Buffing and Boosting phases. My goal was to develop a supplement that was extremely effective but also mild enough to be taken by every woman indefinitely. The HT pill contains a gentle combination of vitamins and nutrients to compliment your hormone levels and <u>does not</u> contain wild amounts of stimulants that may add strain to you adrenal system.

The Buffing Pill (pink)- Works in conjunction with what is happening with your body at this time and with what the HT program prescribes for the Buffing phase regarding fitness and nutrition. Overall, the Buffing pill helps you stay focused and get the progress you are working so relentlessly for during Buffing.

The Boosting Pill (purple)- Works in conjunction with what is happening with your body at this time and with what the HT program prescribes for the Boosting phase regarding fitness and nutrition. Overall, the Boosting supplement is phenomenal for getting over the hump of PMS.

Benefits of the HT Pill:
It reminds you of 4 important keys to success.
1. Pink pill reminds you that you are Buffing. LOSE WEIGHT!
2. Purple pill reminds you that are Boosting. BOOST METABOLISM!
3. You will be reminded of the commitment you made to yourself and your legacy.
4. You will have peace of mind knowing that the Buffing phase gives you what your body needs on a cellular level during that part of your cycle and the same goes for the Boosting phase.

The supplements will work better month after month to create MOMENTUM.
Because the HT Pill works by gradually restoring the body's balance of essential elements, it will usually take a few months to reach a full effect. Often loved ones will begin noting improvements after the first month while you will begin to notice that you feel much better within 2 to 3 months. Sustained well being requires that HT Pill supplementation be continued even after the symptoms of HIF (Hormone Induced Failure) dissipate. The Hormonal Timing Pill will help you stay consistent, and your results will continue to improve the longer you follow the lifestyle.

Other Supplements
After you have a good nutritional base, consider supplementing with other key nutrients:

Protein Supplements (Powders/Bars)-

Protein supplements have been an absolute "Godsend" for me and nearly every one of my private clients. Here's why:

- Speed- I am simply too busy to prepare and eat enough meat, fish, eggs, etc, to fulfill my daily protein requirements. However, I can make and drink a shake in 2 minutes!
- Convenience- I can always have a protein bar in my purse in case I need a quick snack.

NOTE: Some people experience side effects from using popular protein powders such as:
- Upset stomach
- Gas, Bloat
- Diarrhea
- Constipation

In my experience, these side effects occur due to one or more of the following reasons:

1. Overuse! Protein powders and bars are <u>supplements</u>, and are not to be used as the BASE of your diet. Keep your intake of these products to no more than 1-2 servings daily.
2. Sugar Alcohols- low carb, no carb bars and protein drinks often contain sugar alcohols instead of fat or carbs. Be aware that these may cause stomach discomfort (sugar alcohols are the same ingredients used in some laxatives).
3. Artificial Sweeteners- are prevalent in many of the popular protein supplements. They can cause stomach discomfort. I recommend using PURER forms of protein powders to avoid this. They may not taste quite as good but they are so much healthier.
4. Improper hydration- as you consume more protein and become more active you need more water to stay hydrated...so make sure to drink enough water.
5. Not enough greens- You need fiber. If your diet is high on protein and low on green veggies you will have bathroom issues...so make sure to eat your foliage!

Fat burners-

Generally speaking, I do not recommend taking fat burners (stimulant based) for the following reasons:

- They have the potential to cause significant negative effects on your adrenal system. This can lead to numerous future health problems.
- I've never seen anyone experience long-term success from taking them.

- People who use them as a long-term weight solution end up looking and feeling very unhealthy.

If you decide to give them a try, make sure to use them on a limited basis. For instance, one day a week for a little extra kick in your workout. I'm not saying that you should never ever take fat burners. What I am saying is that they are not a healthy long-term solution. In my opinion, they should be used very strategically and never more than 1 or 2 days per week.

L-Glutamine-
- The most abundant amino acid in the body.
- It is vital for muscle maintenance and immune function.
- I recommend it highly for better muscle recovery and prevention of soreness.
- Great for women because of no side effects except excellent hair and nail growth!

NO2 (or products derived from l-arganine)-
- These are some of the newer, most promising supplements on the market.
- They've been shown to increase blood flow, thus increasing nutrient and oxygen availability to cells.
- I recommend the AKG type products that do not contain creatine.
- I have had great fat loss results from using them myself and I have also experienced a noticeable increase in my sexual performance and pleasure.
- For most women, dosing does not need to be as high compared to the general label recommendations. About half the recommended dose works well. (1-2 pills 1-2 times daily vs. 3 pills 3 times daily)
- You MUST take it on an EMPTY stomach. Wait 30-45 min. to eat after (i.e. consume early morning, before lunch, immediately post workout).

Joint supplements-
- I recommend ones that contain glucosamine, chondroitin and hyaluronic acid.
- These are vital for us in order to stay active as we age.
- Help rebuild joint cartilage.
- Prevent inflammation which causes joint pain, damage and stiffness.

Creatine-
Creatine is a great amino acid which provides many benefits in relation to muscle tissue. I use it very strategically depending on my goals. Some of the benefits include:
- Faster muscle recovery so you don't stay sore nearly as long

- Lean muscle growth which will get your metabolism cranking.
- Increased muscle strength- It's much more enjoyable to hit the weights when you feel strong. This increased strength also comes in handy when tackling your daily chores.

However, some people experience side effects from taking creatine such as upset stomach, joint stiffness or pain, and temporary water weight gain.

Don't be afraid to "test" out some supplements yourself. Often times the act of just taking them leads to greater focus and determination to get results. Supplements work both on the physical and mental level. They may just provide you will that little extra push you need to succeed!

Foundation #10: Measure your Success

First off, Get rid of your scale mentality:

We are too often programmed to think we have to weigh a certain amount to be happy. We say to ourselves "If I could only weigh what I did in high school." That thought process can be very defeating; you need to get rid of that scale mentality. **If you are healthy, in shape and happy, who cares how much you weigh?**

The most athletic bodies are often considered overweight if placed on the standard height/weight chart. Why? Because muscle is so dense that the same volume of muscle weighs much more than fat. Muscle also holds about 60 percent more water than fat tissue which adds to the reason why muscular people tend to weigh much more than their "skinny fat" counterparts. So, don't get stuck thinking that you have to be a certain weight. It's more about how you look and perform.

Instead of weight, you should be most concerned about your muscle mass percentage and your body fat percentage, your body composition. How much muscle and fat is on your body? Does it jiggle and wiggle? Or are you firm and tight? To be buff you need to have a high percentage of muscle and a lower amount of body fat. That way you can see the sexy shape of your body that your fat is hiding.

Please also realize that fat not only resides on top of your muscle but INSIDE your muscle. It is marbled in there similar to a rib eye steak. So when you are out of shape and you think your muscles look big, realize that they are not all muscle, there is FAT hiding in them that only consistent EXERCISE and a good diet can melt away.

Measure your success in more ways than numbers

Getting in shape takes patience, consistency and TIME!
If you feel like you aren't getting there fast enough...
You have to find more measurements for your success:

Do you feel a sense of accomplishment?

Are you increasing your weights at the gym?

Are you getting in better shape?

Do you have a an overall better mood?

How do you look?

How do you feel?

Are your rings looser?

Do your muscles feel firmer?

Do you feel more coordinated, agile or flexible?

Do you have more confidence?

Do you have more energy?

Are you learning new things?

Are you being a good example to your kids, family and friends?

Are you inspiring others to make changes themselves?

There is so much more to all of this than your immediate measurable results. You are doing GREAT!!! Keep it up!

As you perform your fitness and diet program, it is smart to record your daily progress toward your goals so that you can track your success...

"BELIEVE that every activity, set, rep, veggie you eat, glass of water you drink, etc... affects every CELL of you body in a positive way forever!"

Nuts and Bolts for ACTION

Success Tool #10: FOUNDATIONS Success Journal

The Foundations Success Journal makes it simple for you to measure your success and incorporate Success Tools #1-9 into your life. Make no mistake, the reason my clients experience such dramatic results is because they use a few simple, very specific foundational principles and they use them RELENTLESSLY! The important thing to understand about every foundational principle is the FACT that you have 100% total control over all of them. You must forget about everything you can't control. If you focus on the millions of things you can't control, you will go crazy and drain your energy on all the wrong thoughts and actions. Every ounce of energy must go into building your Foundations for SUCCESS.

Foundation #1: Realize That You Are In A Battle!
♀ **Success Tool #1- Identify Your HIF Patterns**
- Chart your cycle daily! Always know what c-day you are on.
- Note your weight and water weight (Bloat Factor) daily.
- Journal and be aware of how Hormones effect your body and mind.
- Look back to compare how you felt the previous month on that c-day.

Foundation #2: Hormonal Timing
♀ **Success Tool #2- Buffing and Boosting**
- Always know if you are Buffing or Boosting.
- Stay focused on your goals for that particular phase.

Foundation #3: You Must BELIEVE!
♀ **Success Tool #3- "Doubt Crushers"**
- Have you "truth hammer" always ready to crush doubt. Write it daily as a reminder.
- Believe you can reach your goals and you will!

Foundation #4: PMA- All The Way BABY!
♀ **Success Tool #4- Focus On Solutions**
- Write the solutions to the challenges you face and FOCUS on them!
- Prioritize your "Take Action List" based on importance of what will give you the most results towards reaching your goals.

Foundation #5: Energize Others
♀ **Success Tool #5- The Rally Room**
- Plant "energy seeds" in other's lives and you will soon find exponential energy in your life.
- Who did you energize (encourage) today?

Nuts and Bolts for ACTION

- Utilize the Rally Room for planting your "energy seeds," it is the perfect "Field of Dreams".

Foundation #6: Live With a Legacy Perspective!
♀ **Success Tool #6- The 24 Hour Legacy Test**
- Did you live with a legacy perspective today?
- What did you do today that will produce a <u>positive</u> legacy?

Foundation #7: Momentum! BuffMoJo!
♀ **Success Tool #7- "5 Minute MoJo"**
- List the little things you did today to keep your MoJo. Every moments actions determine your momentum (MoJo).
- Is your momentum headed in the right direction? If not get positive mojo ASAP by using "5 Minute MoJo".

Foundation #8: Plan Of Attack! (POA)
♀ **Success Tool #8- Step By Step Illustrated Exercise Plan**
- Always start your workout with a warm up.
- Note your mood and intensity during your workout.
- Journal your workout so you will see your progress, stay accountable, and have another measurement for success.
- <u>All</u> activity adds up so be sure to count the "extras"!

Foundation #9: Simple Diet and Supplementation
♀ **Success Tool #9- The 5-4-3-2-1 Diet**
- Use the cross off portion tracker to be sure you are getting the right nutrients in your diet daily, remember: KISS!
- Fuel your workouts properly by noting pre and post workout meals.
- Be sure to take your supplements: a multi-vitamin, calcium and The Hormonal Timing Pill for a good nutritional base.

Foundation #10: Measuring Success
♀ **Success Tool #10- Foundations Success Journal**
- Using this journal will help keep you on the RIGHT path towards success.
- Success is not measured in weight loss. Your success is measured by the legacy you leave behind. If you keep a legacy perspective the visual results will follow!
- Remember you are in control of your Body, Life and Legacy!!!

Nuts and Bolts for ACTION

Success Tool #10: Foundations Success Journal (my example)

#1 Chart Cycle C-Day: **25**   Date: **10-27**   Day: **SAT**
Weight: **128**   Bloat Factor 1 - ②- 3

HORMONES
Note Effects: (good or bad)
I feel a little blah! and a bit bloated - not bad
How did I feel last month on this C-day?
I had a cold

#2 Am I Buffing or (Boosting?)

#3 MY "Truth Hammer": **BELIEVE!**
I am building muscle that will BURN FAT!!

#4 PMA "Focus on Solutions"
Take Action List: - for Peace

PRIORITY LEVEL
- 4 ~~Laundry~~
- 1 ~~read Bible - PROVERBS~~
- 2 ~~EDIT Book~~
- 5 ~~Cut Gunner's Hair~~
- 3 ~~Bring in Dry Cleaning~~
- 6 ~~answer e-mails~~

#5 Who did I energize today? (energy seeds)
My son - cheering @ FB game
Julie, Cara & Lisa in the RR!

#6 LEGACY PERSPECTIVE!
In the last day DID YOU?:

Have PMA?	Ⓨ N	Care for YOU	Ⓨ N
Say, "I love you"	Ⓨ N	Work hard	Ⓨ N
Laugh or Smile	Ⓨ N	Eat Well	Ⓨ N
Praise Others	Ⓨ N	*taught Gunner*	
Complain or Yell	Ⓨ N	*to cook soup!*	Y N

#7 The Little Things = MOMENTUM!

Truth. Acts. Habits.	
MY WO	✓
CLEANED	✓
READ BIBLE	✓
CHURRED	✓
3 GREENS!	✓
WORKED	✓

"5 MIN MoJo"
1 - ☐ Drink 10oz. H₂O
2 - ☐ MARCH 1 min.
3 - ☑ 5 FULL breaths
4 - ☐ STRETCH 1 min.
5 - ☑ Eat a GREEN!

#8 POA warm up! **7:30 r-bike**
mode & min.
Mood: 😄 😢 😐   Time: **1:00pm - 2:10**
Intensity: ① 2 - 3

Exercises: Weight x Reps Set 1 Set 2 Set 3 Set 4

Exercises	Set 1	Set 2	Set 3	Set 4
Bench Press	45x20	95x10	135x6 x2	
Incline Hammer	80x6	100x6	120x6	
Incline Flys	30x10	40x6 x 2 sets	1PR!	
Tri Extension	40x10	50x6 x2		
Tri Pushdowns	90x10 x 3 sets			
Knee ups - R-chair	40	35	25	

Any PB's? **Yes I-flys!** Sore? **Back - lats**
Daily Core: **knee ups, CATS, vacuums**
"BuffMotherobics" **20 min intervals**
or Other Cardio: **on elliptical**
EXTRAS? shop walk (clean) play (sex)

#9 The 5 - 4 - 3 - 2 - 1 Diet (K.I.S.S.)
R R R R R
C C C C
F F F
G G G
T
Supplements:
ND₂ am - Multi & Cal
Joint, Fishoil

HT Pill? Ⓨ N
wwwwwwwww

Pre-WO Meal: *oatmeal & boca burger*
Post-WO Meal: *protein shake w/ blueberries*

Thoughts / Notes / Prayers:
I am proud I got it done today. I sought PEACE today and had it! COOL! Gunner won his game too!! I have to drink more water tommorrow & cut Gun's hair!

Nuts and Bolts for ACTION

112

Hello —

    I just wanted to say "thanks" for reading MY book!! I am beyond excited to finally have it in your hands. I know it may not be perfect, but I wrote it with LOVE! I really hope something I've shared in these pages has helped you.

    My faith in Jesus Christ has been the KEY reason for my success. Without it I'd be lost! He has given me the courage, strength and determination to go after my DREAMS!

    Please allow yourself to <u>BELIEVE</u> you can live your dreams!!

Love, your new friend,

Michelle Berger
— Buff Mother! —

Nuts and Bolts for ACTION

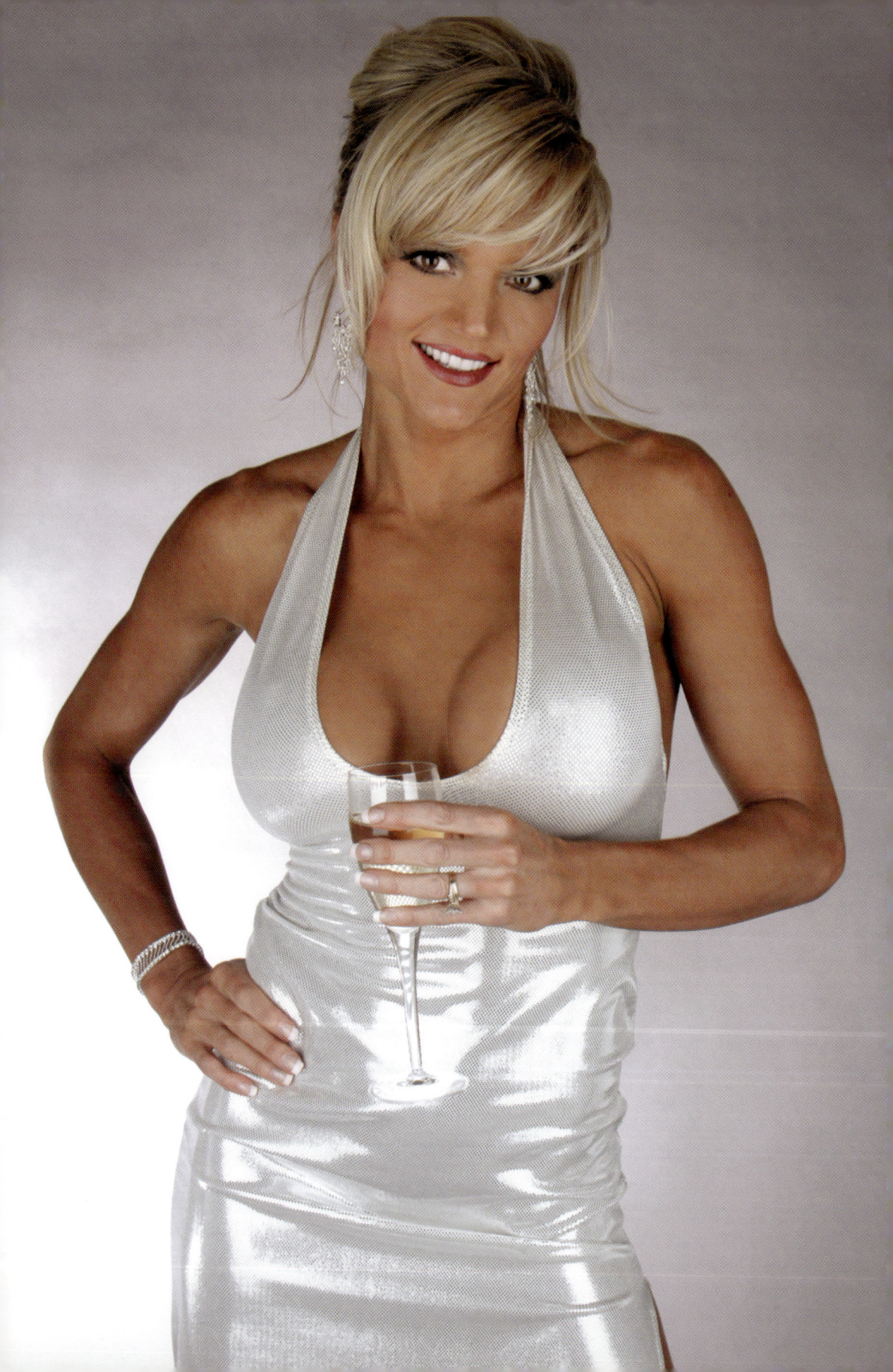

BONUS section

10 Keys to GREAT Hormonal Timing SEX!

Hormonal Timing will dramatically improve your sex life!!!

For the sake of this section, I'm going to assume that you are married, in love with your husband and have a strong desire to partner with him for awesome sex. Also, I realize that the recipe for great sex is very complex and goes way beyond the physical. That being said, your body is your vehicle for sex. Time for an analogy; Think back to the worst car you've ever driven. It was slow, unresponsive, uncomfortable, you can fill in the rest... Now, imagine going from that to the best car you've driven. Wow, it was a radically different driving experience wasn't it? Hormonal Timing will turn your body into a great sexual vehicle. **Here are 10 reasons why, how, etc...**

1) **Lower BODY FAT-** Within 30 days of starting the HT lifestyle, your body fat will begin to melt away. This will give you more confidence in bed. You will want to buy some sexy lingerie or be naked more often as this confidence develops. This will be enough to create some sparks but it's only the starting point. Our mission is an inferno!!

2) **Muscle Tone-** The strength training component will help you develop some muscle tone. Remember, muscle tone is the only thing that separates you from your youth. This muscle tone is a turn on for your partner but even more of a turn on for you! A stronger body is critical for sexual performance and endurance which leads to incredible orgasms!!

3) **Knowledge is power!** Chart your libido for the anticipation of mind blowing sex. Your Hormone fluctuations have a HUGE impact on your natural state of arousal at any given time of the month. Charting your libido is a very powerful tool for great sex.

Patterns will develop- You will begin to see very specific sexual arousal tendencies almost immediately as you chart your hormones. As you progress in your physical fitness, you will become acutely aware of your "high" times because they will be unmistakable.

Share this information with your husband. I keep a BIG calendar on my bedroom wall that notes which c-day I am on. This helps me keep tabs on where I'm at hormonally...and trust me your DH (internet jargon: Dear Husband) pays attention. It started off with him wanting to know when TOM was coming, (I think he just wanted to know which days he'd be "shut down.") Then as my charting got more in depth, he started to prepare for when I'd be ovulating in order to really capitalize on my super charged hormonal state. It's amazing how creative he is during this "high" time. He also knows that on day 22 he needs to disappear completely! He honestly wants to work with my hormones and utilize them to his advantage!! It's turned into a fun little game with us and has added an incredible dimension to that part of our lives.

4) **How to Chart your libido:**
Things to chart so that you know your sexy side:
Responsiveness- both physically and mentally
Thought patterns
Romantic thoughts
Yearn for physical contact
Your desire to please your husband
Your desire to be pleased
ETC...

BONUS: **Hormonal Timing SEX**

You could do a human experiment...shoot to have sex as often as possible this month and chart your findings.

From your charting results do the following activity to apply HORMONAL TIMING SEX:

- Figure out at least 2 days a month that you will be the sexual aggressor (for example good ones I've found are between c-day 6 and 17)
- Share at least 2 days with your husband a month that you are responsive, but you want him to want you!! For instance day 13 just prior to ovulation or day 27 or 28 just prior to your period

My Hormonal Timing Sex Chart:

C-Day	Physical	Libido
1, 2, 3	Period	Usually a NO GO!
4, 5, 6	Low hormones	A bit low
7, 8, 9, 10, 11, 12	Feel good	Confident and ON!
(13, 14, 15)	Approx. ovulation	One really good day, the others may be bloated and some pain
18, 19, 20	Feel decent	Responsive but not aggressive
21, 22, 23	Feel like crying	Hold me, kiss me, and we'll see
24, 25, 26	Tired	Responsive, but don't wait until 11pm to approach me
27, 28	High hormones	May be HOT! Chocolate cravings may be SEX cravings in reality

5) **Use BuffMother Psychology**

As a reminder, success in anything starts in your mind. You can use the mental exercises previously discussed to greatly enhance your sex life.

The "mental side" of SEX:
- Believe that you can have an incredible sex life.
- Choose a powerful affirmation "truth hammer" to crush any doubt the instant it enters your mind.
- PMA- Have a great attitude about sex. Forget the past if necessary and determine to create a positive outlook about sex.
- Use the "focus on solutions" exercise to create and maintain a PMA.
- Remember, You are the "Fixer" in your life.

6) **Create positive momentum**- It's the little things that will create and/or destroy positive momentum. Apply the BuffMoJo strategy to your sex life. Sparking you sexual side little by little can build you sexual momentum into a FIRE!

Spark your SEX MOJO

How many times can you "hit it" with each item on the list below?
- 🔥 Touch your husband
- 🔥 Kiss his lips
- 🔥 Kiss his neck
- 🔥 Kiss his hand
- 🔥 Kiss his neck
- 🔥 Grab him
- 🔥 Hug him
- 🔥 Say something sexy to him
- 🔥 Say "I love you" in a sexy way
- 🔥 Look at him lustfully
- 🔥 Tell him you want him

HAVE FUN WITH IT!!

7) Take the Hormonal Timing Pill

You will feel a difference quickly, but the best results will take time to develop. You need to take them consistently and believe in the lifestyle. Buff, Boost, Buff, Boost for the rest of your life.

8) Additional Supplementation may help.

I have recently noticed a sudden surge the in the intensity of my, excuse me, "O's" after taking a particular NO2 formulation. It has helped in many other key areas as well. In fact, my results have been dramatic enough that I have decided to add this to my product line upon completing a little more research.

9) Apply the Exponential Energy principle

I know that when it comes to sex, this can be very difficult. However, if you are willing to take the first step and give sexual energy to your husband, you will be richly rewarded.

Please just try it for 30 days. You will be blown away by what happens. The rewards you experience will go way beyond sex. I promise.

10) God designed us to have and enjoy great sex!

He made women beautiful, gorgeous, and sexy for a reason. He gave us all the tools to be great lovers and to be the objects of our husband's desires. There is nothing wrong with being sexy as long as our motives are pure! What I'm trying to say is: Give yourself permission to be sexy!!

BONUS: Hormonal Timing SEX

Appendixes

A. Success Tool #1-Identify HIF Patterns

B. Starting Statistics, Measurements, and Pictures

C. Guideline for Progression of Workouts

D. Sample Diet Menu

E. Success Tool #10-Foundations Success Journal

F. Other Resources and Products by BuffMother!

Appendix A: Success Tool #1- Identify HIF Patterns (chart cycle)

C-day Date	Weight	Bloat	Mood	Focus	Stress	Energy	Pain	Hunger	Strength	Sleep	Libido	Other
1												
2												
3												
4												
5												
6												
7												
8												
9												
10												
11												
12												
13												
14												
15												
16												
17												
18												
19												
20												
21												
22												
23												
24												
25												
26												
27												
28												
29												
30												
31												
32												

Appendix

Appendix B- Starting statistics, measurements, and pictures

Today's Date:_____ height:_____ weight:_____ age:_____
Today's cycle day-_____

Please list the following measurements:
_____ Bust (around breasts the biggest part)
_____ Chest- relaxed (just under armpits above breasts with arms down at your sides)
_____ Chest- flexed back and chest (just under armpits with arms down at your sides)
_____ Waist- relaxed (the smallest part)
_____ Waist-sucked in (the smallest part)
_____ Hips (the largest part of your butt)
_____ Shoulders (around the outside of your shoulders with your arms at sides)
_____ Biceps (relaxed at midpoint of upper arm)
_____ Biceps (flexed at midpoint of upper arm)
_____ Thigh-mid (about 8" above knee cap)
_____ Thigh- upper (about 12" above knee cap)
_____ Calf (about 7" below knee joint)

Body Fat- An optional measurement...the scale or hand held body fat measurements are not accurate, but may be a tiny help when used as a baseline to measure progress. I'd suggest using an experienced trainer at a local gym to measure you with calipers. A 3 site test is adequate; however you can do up to 7 sites. Be sure that you get measured by the same person each time and ask for the results to include each site's caliper millimeter(mm) measurement along with the body fat calculation. I often times don't figure the % just look for the caliper measurements to go down.

Progress Pictures- Aim to produce photos that will be most comparable with the next set of progress photos you take. Photo are best taken in good lighting (during the day), from the same distances and angles, on a light background and in the same clothing (bikini if possible). It is best for you to take following poses* all **full body**:
1. straight on arms at sides
2. straight on arms up and flexed
3. from behind with arms at sides
4. behind with arms up flexing biceps
5. from the side
6. model or movie star pose- have fun!

*You can do them both relaxed and flexed. Have fun and SMILE!

Measure your PROGRESS:
Take your measurements, stats and photos again. Don't wait until you are PERFECT, but do it along the way to see if what you are doing is working. It is best to take the photos no more often than in 2 week periods. 6-12 weeks is the best timeframe to see visible change.

Appendix C- Guideline for the next "level" of workouts.

I generally deal with 4 levels of fitness programs: Beginner, Experienced, Advanced and Elite. Once you progress past the Beginner workouts you will want to utilize an Experienced workout calendar similar to this:

Experienced Buffing and Boosting workout calendar:

	MON	TUE	WED	THU	FRI	SAT	SUN
Week 1	Lift upper body Intervals	Lift lower body	Intervals	Lift upper body Intervals	Lift lower body	Intervals	off
Week 2	Lift upper body Intervals	Lift lower body	Intervals	Lift upper body Intervals	Lift lower body	Intervals	off

	MON	TUE	WED	THU	FRI	SAT	SUN
Week 3	Lift upper body	Lift lower body	Intervals	Lift upper body	Lift lower body	Intervals	off
Week 4	Lift upper body	Lift lower body	Intervals	Lift upper body	Lift lower body	Intervals	off

Experienced Intervals or "BuffMotherobics!"

"**Even Minute Intervals**": every min that starts with an even number push it hard, recover at a slower pace during the odd min. Start hard minutes at min #4 and the last hard min #16. Here is the breakdown:

Min 1-3 min. warm up
Min 4-1 min. hard
Min 5-1 min. easy
Min 6-1 min. hard
Min 7-1 min. easy
Min 8-1 min. hard
Min 9-1 min. easy
Min 10-1 min. hard

Min 11-1 min. easy
Min 12-1 min. hard
Min 13-1 min. easy
Min 14-1 min. hard
Min 15-1 min. easy
Min 16-1 min. hard
Min 17-20 3min. easy cool down

This is 20 min total includes 7 hard minutes!! Way to go!
*If you don't feel exhausted by the end, increase the intensity of the hard and/or easy minutes rather than adding time.

Appendix D: Sample diet menu (Buffing Phase) …just some ideas for what and when to eat during Buffing.

Goal Intake for the day: 5P-3C-3F-3G

Wake-up: Water, and any supplements that need to be taken on an empty tummy

Meal #1: 3 eggs and whole grain toast (you can take this to go by eating hard boiled eggs and making your toast as you go out the door, I have also done scrambled eggs in a baggy and refrigerate for use later)
PFC

Meal #2: 3-4oz. turkey or chicken and Brussels sprouts- these are great for snacking on at your desk (I cook mine in the microwave in a ceramic bowl covered with a plate 1 TBS water for 5 min. uncover and let cool for 5 mins.)
   A great time to take the rest of your supplements.
PG

Meal #3: 3-4oz. tuna or salmon salad (fish+tsp. miracle whip+pickle relish) on celery or salmon on celery
PFG

Meal #4: pre-workout (1.5 hours before workout) Whey protein powder in water and apple (may want to peel it to prevent tummy discomfort) or oat meal
P C

Meal #5: post workout (take your l-glutamine if you didn't in the am or if you're extra sore) eat as soon after your workout as possible.
   4 oz. beef meal (burger patty, taco meat, roast) or STEAK
   A BIG salad (greens- romaine or leaf lettuce, cucumber, spinach, peppers, mushrooms, olives/nuts/dressing (as an accent))
   1 C- fruit, corn, rice, blueberries or a very small dessert item-125cals
PCFGG

Snack Ideas-
In a pinch you can use these items for P's (protein)- turkey jerky, turkey salami, a ready to drink protein shake (no carb), protein bar, etc.
Guilt fee carb snack- blueberries
Guilt free fat snack- sunflower seeds in the shell
Free snacks (don't count)- any extra greens and herbal tea (some of my favorites: cucumbers, brussel sprouts, asparagus, chamomile tea, peppermint tea, chai tea)

If you miss a meal combine your protein servings at the next meal and forget about the missed C, G or F. You can eat it later if you are starving. Listen to your body!

Appendix E: Success Tool # 10 - Foundations Success Journal

#1 Chart Cycle   C-Day:_____   Date:_____   Day:_____

HORMONES

Weight:_____   Bloat Factor 1 – 2 – 3

Note Effects: (good or bad)

How did I feel last month on this C-day?

#2 Am I *Buffing* or *Boosting*?

#3 MY "Truth Hammer": **BELIEVE!**
_____

#4 PMA "Focus on Solutions"
Take Action List:

PRIORITY LEVEL
- ☐ _____
- ☐ _____
- ☐ _____
- ☐ _____
- ☐ _____
- ☐ _____

#5 Who did I energize today?
(energy seeds)
_____
_____

#6 LEGACY PERSPECTIVE!
In the last day DID YOU?:

Have PMA?	Y N	Care for YOU	Y N
Say, "I love you"	Y N	Work hard	Y N
Laugh or Smile	Y N	Eat Well	Y N
Praise Others	Y N		Y N
Complain or Yell	Y N		Y N

#7 The Little Things = MOMENTUM!

The little things I did today

"5 MIN MoJo"
1- ☐ Drink 10oz. H₂O
2- ☐ MARCH 1 min.
3- ☐ 5 FULL breaths
4- ☐ STRETCH 1 min.
5- ☐ Eat a GREEN!

#8 POA   warm up!
mode & min._____

Mood: 😁 😢 😐   Time:_____
Intensity: 1 - 2 - 3
Weight x Reps

Exercises:	Set 1	Set 2	Set 3	Set 4

Any PB's?	Sore?

Daily Core:

"BuffMotherobics"
or Other Cardio:

EXTRAS?   shop   walk   clean   play   sex

#9 The 5 - 4 - 3 - 2 - 1 Diet (K.I.S.S.)

P P P P P   Supplements:
C C C C   _____
F F F   _____
G G ___
T   HT Pill? Y N
W W W W W W W W W W W W
Pre-WO Meal:_____
Post-WO Meal:_____

Thoughts / Notes / Prayers:

Appendix F: Other resources and products by BuffMother!

The Web-site...www.BuffMother.com
- The Official HOME of Team BuffMother!
- Connect with me through my Daily Blog, My story, My Gallery, My Testimony and through my hang out...the Rally Room
- Join Team BuffMother for free and you will so you can be a part of the revolution which entitles you to many benefits.
- Be inspired by other women just like you through the featured Success Stories, the Team BuffMother Gallery and in the Rally Room.
- Enjoy many free articles and fun products: books, customized plans, supplements, shirts and more!

The Rally Room-

There is a place you can go where the sole purpose is to use your gifts to help other women. The power that is released in that place is indescribable! This place is located online and is called the Rally Room. It is a secure, women only, part of www.BuffMother.com. Everyone brings their own brand of positive energy to the team and they receive an explosion of positive energy in return. You can never out give this team!

Customized Hormonal Timing Plan-

I have made every effort to make this book as simple and "user friendly" as possible. My goal was to spell everything out in such a way that anyone could use the information to design their very own Customized Hormonal Timing Plan. However, I know that many women would rather not go through the "Do It Yourself" process. Instead, they would rather just have everything lined out for them. They say, "just tell me what to do and when to do it!" If this describes you, then you might want to consider having me design a program for you. This is the most turnkey approach to living the Hormonal Timing Lifestyle because I will tell you what to do and when to do it based on your individual needs. I'll take out all the "guesswork" so you can focus your energy on taking action! You can access your own plan at www.BuffMother.com.

The Hormonal Timing Pill (Buffing and Boosting pills)-

As you can imagine, I highly recommend taking The Hormonal Timing Pill on a daily basis in conjunction with a multivitamin and calcium supplementation. The Hormonal Timing Pill (Buffing/Boosting Pills) are designed to complement your body chemistry and goals as you progress through your Buffing and Boosting phase of Hormonal Timing.

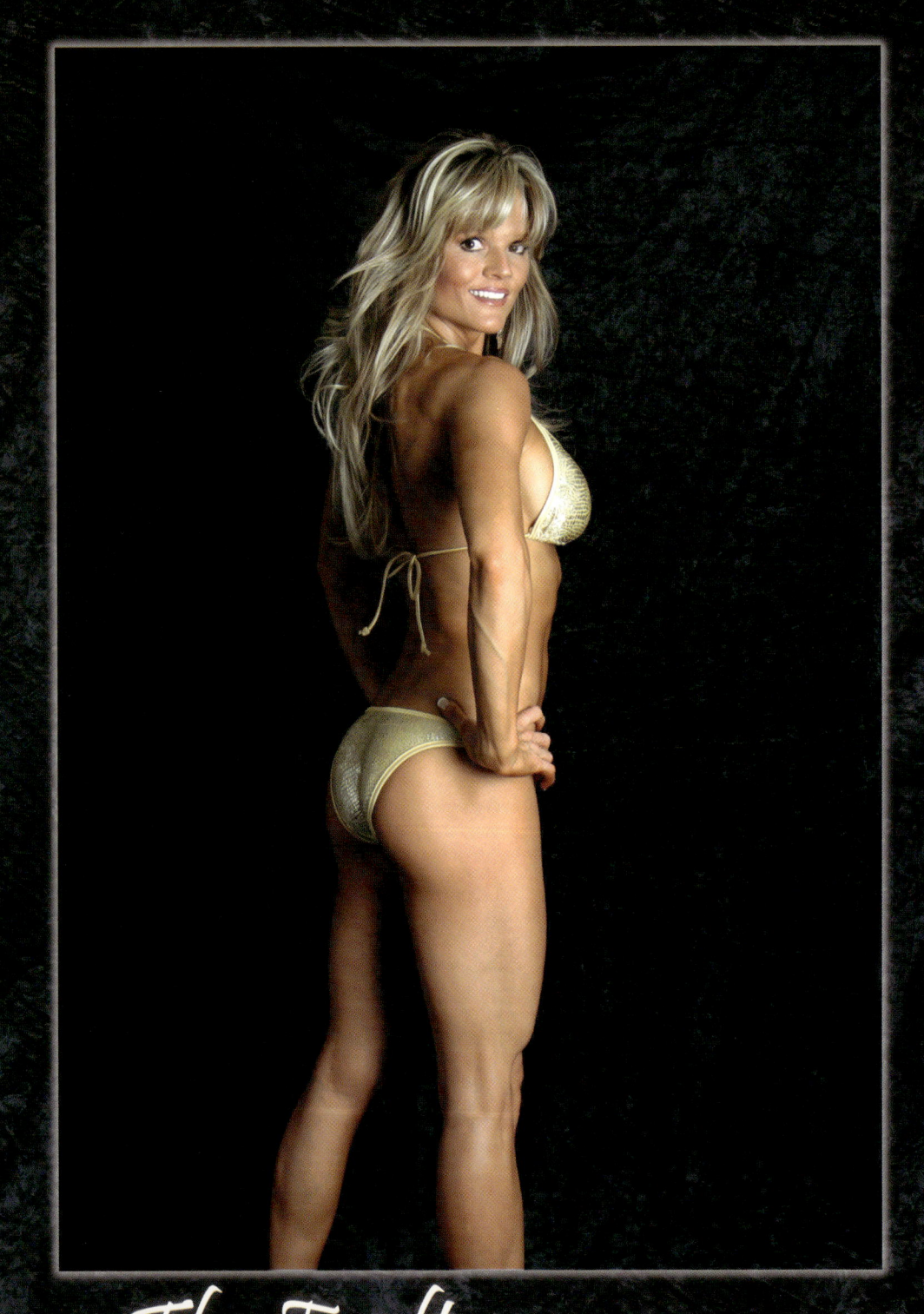

The End!
...or is this just the Beginning?

Has this book inspired you?
Did you have a "light bulb moment"?
Have you changed the way you approach your fitness, diet, or life?
Please share your thoughts!!

Do you have a success story?
No one has a story like yours!
You can inspire others with your success!
Please share your story!!

You have the power to inspire others with your words. Please share with ME, how this book has affected you and those around you!

Feel free to e-mail me: michelle@buffmother.com
or you can send me a note by mail:

BuffMother! attn: Michelle
902A. S. Walton Blvd. Ste.1-286
Bentonville, AR 72712

Don't forget to keep your motivation and energy high by connecting to
TEAM BuffMother! online at www.BuffMother.com